高职高专院校专业基础课纸数融合系列教材

供临床医学、护理、助产、药学、影像、检验、口腔医学、康复等专业使用

U0166069

医护英语

YIHU YINGYU

主　编　张　莹　郑丽红

副主编　李婉瑄　牛晓伟　郭鸣鹃

编　者　（以姓氏笔画为序）

王仙凤　上海东海职业技术学院

牛晓伟　上海东海职业技术学院

许艳婷　漳州卫生职业学院

苏小青　上海东海职业技术学院

李晓红　上海东海职业技术学院

李清花　上海东海职业技术学院

李婉瑄　广州卫生职业技术学院

张　莹　辽宁医药职业学院

陈琳宁　漳州卫生职业学院

郑丽红　漳州卫生职业学院

倪盈盈　上海东海职业技术学院

郭鸣鹃　漳州卫生职业学院

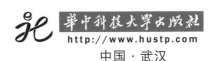

华中科技大学出版社

http://www.hustp.com

中国·武汉

内 容 简 介

本书为高职高专院校专业基础课纸数融合系列教材。

本书参考高等学校英语应用能力考试大纲,针对高职高专学生的需求和学力基础等具体情况,充分利用二语习得的相关理论进行编写。全书共分为12个单元,每个单元围绕一个特定的主题(挂号、门诊、药房、住院等)编写,每一主题都贴近学生的学习、生活。此外,书中穿插大量与教学内容有关的数字资源,包括PPT、课文和对话部分音频及习题答案等丰富的形式,可以更为有效地激发学生的学习热情和兴趣。

本书可供高职专科、成人专科学生学习,亦可供具有一定英语基础知识的社会人员自主学习。

图书在版编目(CIP)数据

医护英语/张莹,郑丽红主编.—武汉:华中科技大学出版社,2021.1(2025.2重印)
ISBN 978-7-5680-6867-3

Ⅰ.①医… Ⅱ.①张… ②郑… Ⅲ.①医学-英语 Ⅳ.①R

中国版本图书馆 CIP 数据核字(2021)第 017392 号

医护英语
Yihu Yingyu

张 莹 郑丽红 主编

策划编辑:史燕丽
责任编辑:史燕丽 张 萌
封面设计:原色设计
责任校对:李 弋
责任监印:周治超
出版发行:华中科技大学出版社(中国·武汉)　　　电话:(027)81321913
　　　　　武汉市东湖新技术开发区华工科技园　　　邮编:430223
录　排:华中科技大学惠友文印中心
印　刷:武汉市籍缘印刷厂
开　本:889mm×1194mm　1/16
印　张:8.25
字　数:256千字
版　次:2025 年 2 月第 1 版第 2 次印刷
定　价:49.90元

网络增值服务使用说明

欢迎使用华中科技大学出版社医学资源网yixue.hustp.com

1.教师使用流程

（1）登录网址：http://yixue.hustp.com（注册时请选择教师用户）

（2）审核通过后，您可以在网站使用以下功能：

管理学生

建立课程　　　　　　　　布置作业

下载教学
资源　　　　　　教师　　　　　查询学生学习
记录等

2.学员使用流程

建议学员在PC端完成注册、登录、完善个人信息的操作。

（1）PC端学员操作步骤

①登录网址：http://yixue.hustp.com（注册时请选择普通用户）

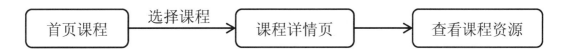

②查看课程资源

如有学习码，请在个人中心-学习码验证中先验证，再进行操作。

首页课程　—选择课程→　课程详情页　→　查看课程资源

（2）手机端扫码操作步骤

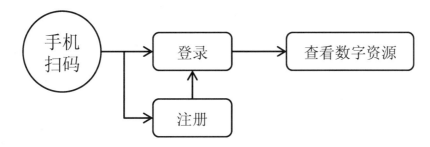

习近平总书记在十九大报告中提出"中国特色社会主义进入新时代"。新时代促进中国社会飞速发展，从而吸引了越来越多的外国人来到中国学习、工作和生活，推动了越来越多的中国人走出国门寻找就业机会。简单的基础英语交际技能已无法满足新时代背景下社会对于人才具有"复合能力"的需求。为了满足这一需求，培养应用型、综合型、国际化的医护人才，我们编写了《医护英语》这本教材。

本教材主要供医药类高职院校各专业学生及在职医疗卫生人员或对医护英语感兴趣爱好者使用，是贯通公共基础英语与专业英语之间的桥梁教材。本书以"工学为主，能力为本"的职业教育理念为编写原则，从医护岗位需求出发，注重语言在不同岗位工作场景下的实际运用，以帮助学生掌握未来工作中所需的医护英语基本知识和技能为目标，从而实现理论与实践的无缝对接。

本教材以医院为背景，内容涵盖相关科室日常医护岗位所需要的专业英语基本知识、工作用语以及会话用语，使学生能就医护话题用英语在医患、护患、医护之间进行交流，撰写与医护工作相关的文书，如询问病史、填写病历、汇报病情等。同时，本教材还为学生提供了很多拓展知识，为学生进一步提升自己的知识水平以及后续专业英语的学习打下坚实的基础。

由于作者水平有限，疏漏之处在所难免，恳请广大读者和同仁批评指正，以帮助我们再版时改进。

编 者
2021 年 1 月

目　录

MULU

Unit 1 Registration and Making an Appointment

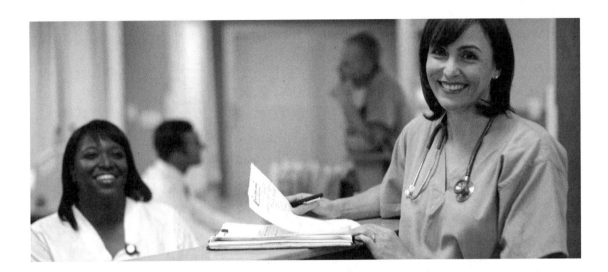

扫码看
PPT

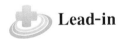 **Lead-in**

In China, the first step of visiting a doctor is registration. People can simply show up at a hospital, register with and see a doctor without making an appointment. However, in western countries, no preset appointment will not be accepted. In recent years, however, more and more Chinese people have been encouraged to register online or by telephone if there is no emergency.

Thinking & Talking

1. Which way do you prefer when you need to see a doctor? Why?

2. What should you take with when you see a doctor?

Focus Listening

扫码听
对话1

Conversation 1

Directions: *Mr. Smith is making a call to register at a hospital. Here is a conversation between* <u>*Mr. Smith and a nurse*</u>. *Choose the best answer for each of the following questions.*

1. Why can't Mr. Smith register right now? _____.

A. Because of the power cut

Note

B. Because of lack of ID card

C. Because of the system failure

2. Is this the first visit for Mr. Smith? _____.

A. Yes，it is　　　　　　　　B. No，it isn't　　　　　　　C. It is unmentioned

3. How will Mr. Smith register this time? _____.

A. Register online　　　　　B. Go to registration office　　C. On the call

4. Which department did Mr. Smith register with? _____.

A. Neurology Department　　B. Stomatology Department　C. Gastroenterology Department

5. Which card is NOT necessary for registration? _____.

A. ID card　　　　　　　　B. Credit card　　　　　　　C. Insurance card

New Words & Expressions

扫码听
单词

registration [ˌredʒɪ'streɪʃən]	n. 挂号，注册
department [dɪ'paːtmənt]	n. 科室，部门
appointment [ə'pɔɪntmənt]	n. 预约，约定
insurance [ɪn'ʃʊərəns]	n. 保险
neurology [ˌnjʊə'rɒlədʒɪ]	n. 神经病学
stomatology [ˌstəʊmə'tɒlədʒɪ]	n. 口腔学
gastroenterology ['gæstrəʊˌentə'rɒlədʒɪ]	n. 胃肠病学

Conversation 2

Directions： *Mr. Lin works oversea in Britain，now he is calling to make an appointment. Listen to the conversation and decide whether the following statements are true（T）or false（F）.*

（　）1. Mr. Lin has never seen Dr. Johnson.

（　）2. Mr. Lin feels uncomfortable on his leg.

（　）3. There are some red spots that make Mr. Lin feels itchy.

（　）4. Mr. Lin will see the doctor at 8：00 a. m.，Tuesday.

New Words & Expressions

physical checkup	体检
locate [ləʊ'keɪt]	v. 定位，查找
spot [spɒt]	n. 斑点
itchy ['ɪtʃɪ]	adj. 发痒的
urgent care	急救
available [ə'veɪləbl]	adj. 可获得的，有空的
convenient [kən'viːnɪənt]	adj. 方便的，适当的

Group Discussion & Role Playing

Note

1. Work in pairs. Suppose a patient is at the registration office. Make a conversation between a nurse and a patient about how to make a registration.

2. Display the conversation you've made.

3. After one group finishes the performance, others make comments.

Intensive Reading

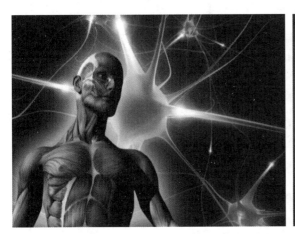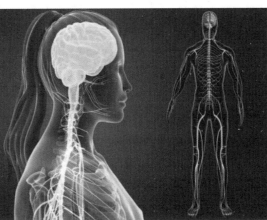

Human Body Systems

Our body consists of a number of biological systems that carry out specific functions for everyday living. Understanding these systems helps us know how the body functions and why keeping healthy is important for our life.

Integumentary System

The integumentary system acts as a barrier to protect us against bacteria and viruses. It also functions to balance body temperature and eliminate waste through perspiration. In addition to skin, the integumentary system includes hair and nails.

Respiratory System

The respiratory system involves in the process of breathing. The primary organs in this process are the lungs, which exchange oxygen for carbon dioxide.

Circulatory System

The circulatory system is a network consisting of the heart, blood and blood vessels. This network provides the cells with nutrients and oxygen, and removes waste products. Our diet and exercise habits may affect our circulatory system.

Musculoskeletal System

The human musculoskeletal system is an organ system that relates to the muscles and the skeleton of the body. It provides support, stability and movement to the body.

Digestive System

The digestive system consists of organs that break down food, absorb nutrients, and expel waste. Most digestive organs form a long, continuous tube called the gastrointestinal tract. The rest of the organs like liver and pancreas are called accessory organs.

Endocrine System

The vital function of the endocrine system is the production and regulation of hormones. Most endocrine disorders occur due to either too much or too little hormone, which include diabetes,

Note

hyperthyroidism and hypothyroidism.

Nervous System

The nervous system is a complex network which sends signals round the body. Structurally, it is made up of the central nervous system(CNS) and the peripheral nervous system(PNS).

Reproductive System

The major function of the reproductive system is to reproduce and generate offspring. Abnormal hormone secretion and other problems in this region frequently affect fertility.

Urinary System

The urinary system keeps our body healthy by removing dangerous waste products from our blood and expelling them from our body in the form of urine. The waste liquid filtered out by the kidneys is stored in the bladder until the body expels it.

New Words & Expressions

integumentary [ɪnˌtegjʊ'mentərɪ]	adj. 外皮的
bacteria [bæk'tɪərɪə]	n. 细菌
eliminate [ɪ'lɪmɪneɪt]	v. 消除,清除
perspiration [ˌpɜːspə'reɪʃən]	n. 汗水,流汗
in addition to	除……之外(还有,也)
respiratory ['respərətərɪ]	adj. 呼吸的
involve [ɪn'vɒlv]	v. 参加,包含
organ ['ɔːgən]	n. 器官
oxygen ['ɒksɪdʒən]	n. 氧气
circulatory [ˌsɜːkjʊ'leɪtərɪ]	adj. 血液循环的
vessel ['vesəl]	n. 脉管,血管
musculoskeletal [ˌmʌskjʊləʊ'skelɪtəl]	adj. 肌(与)骨骼的
stability [stə'bɪlətɪ]	n. 稳定性
digestive [daɪ'dʒestɪv]	adj. 消化的
break down	分解,损坏
expel [ɪk'spel]	v. 驱逐
gastrointestinal [ˌgæstrəʊɪn'testɪnəl]	adj. 胃肠的
pancreas ['pæŋkrɪəs]	n. 胰腺
accessory [ək'sesərɪ]	adj. 附属的,辅助的
endocrine ['endəʊkrɪn]	adj. 内分泌的
hormone ['hɔːməʊn]	n. 激素,荷尔蒙
diabetes [ˌdaɪə'biːtiːz]	n. 糖尿病
hyperthyroidism [ˌhaɪpə'θaɪrɔɪdɪzəm]	n. 甲状腺功能亢进
hypothyroidism [ˌhaɪpəʊ'θaɪrɔɪdɪzəm]	n. 甲状腺功能减退
central nervous system(CNS)	中枢神经系统
peripheral nervous system(PNS)	周围神经系统
reproductive [ˌriːprə'dʌktɪv]	adj. 生殖的,再生的
secretion [sɪ'kriːʃən]	n. 分泌,分泌物

扫码听
单词

fertility [fəˈtɪlətɪ]	n. 生育力
urinary [ˈjʊərɪnərɪ]	adj. 尿的，泌尿的
bladder [ˈblædə(r)]	n. 膀胱

Exercises

Exercise 1. Decide whether the following statements are true (T) or false (F) according to the text.

(   ) 1. Integumentary system is a protector that can defend our body against bacteria and viruses.

(   ) 2. Your lifestyle cannot affect your circulatory system.

(   ) 3. The digestive system consists of organs that enable our body to break down and absorb food.

(   ) 4. Endocrine diseases are always caused by abnormal hormone secretion.

(   ) 5. The urinary system keeps us healthy by filtering out dangerous waste.

Exercise 2. Fill in the blanks with the words given below, changing the form if necessary.

| eliminate | digestive | circulatory | involve |
| fertility | expel | organ | bladder |

1. Drinking too much wine will increase the risk of _____ diseases.

2. This medicine claims to _____ my eye pain.

3. Parents should _____ themselves in their child's education.

4. Improving lifestyle is a good way to prevent _____ diseases.

5. Bladder and kidney are important _____ of urinary system.

Exercise 3. Translate the following Chinese sentences into English.

1. 她的咳嗽是由支气管炎引起的。

2. 糖尿病在肥胖人群中是一种常见疾病。

3. 神经系统不仅包括中枢神经系统，还有周围神经系统。

4. 消化系统的主要功能是分解食物、吸收营养。

5. 为了放松，他深吸了一口气，然后慢慢呼气。

Learning More

Ⅰ. Affixes & Roots of Medical Terms

Affixes & Roots	Chinese	More Words
bio-	生命，生物	biology 生物学；biopsy 活组织检查
-ology	学科，科目	neurology 神经学；stomatology 口腔学
respire(a)-	呼吸	respirator 呼吸器；respiration 呼吸
gastro-	胃的	gastrointestinal 胃肠的；gastroscopy 胃镜检查
hyper-	高于，超过	hypertension 高血压；hyperthyroidism 甲状腺功能亢进

Note

Match the English expressions with the right Chinese phrases.

1. gastroscopy   A. 高血压

2. respiration   B. 生物学家

3. hypertension   C. 胃镜检查

4. biologist   D. 神经病学

5. neurology   E. 呼吸

Ⅱ. Vocabulary Expansion

Match the Chinese phrases with the right English expressions.

A. break down	B. function	C. perspiration
D. eliminate	E. bacteria	F. blood vessels
G. lung	H. appointment	I. registration
J. department	K. secretion	L. reproductive system

1. (　　)流汗   (　　)科室

2. (　　)分泌   (　　)细菌

3. (　　)功能   (　　)肺

4. (　　)分解   (　　)挂号

5. (　　)生殖系统   (　　)血管

Practical Writing

Appointment Record(就诊预约单)

就诊预约单通常为医疗机构登记患者就诊预约信息的表格,应包含以下内容。

1. 患者的个人基本信息,包括姓名、性别、年龄、联系方式、医保信息等。

2. 患者预约的具体信息,包括日期、时间、预约的问诊医生等。

3. 标明初诊或是复诊,以作出相关的就诊提示。

4. 就诊原因说明,以方便医生有效地作出问诊安排。

Sample

Appointment Record	
Full name：Liu Mei	Gender：☑ F □ M
Birth date：Nov. 10，1984	
Phone：158××××××××	
Insurance card No.：00189	
Date：Oct. 9，Wednesday	Time：3：00 p.m.
Preferred doctor：Dr. Johnson	
Is this your first visit to our hospital?	
☑ Yes □ No	
Reasons for visit：Have a recheck on her backache.	

Exercise

Complete the following form according to the information given below.

【张鹏,男,1975 年 9 月 11 日出生,联系方式为 178××××××××,医保卡号为 100456。过去一周由于熬夜加班常感眼睛干涩酸痛。首次预约 6 月 18 日(星期四)上午 9 点,到诊所向 Daniel 医生求诊。】

Appointment Record

Full name：   Gender：□ F   □ M

Birth date：

Phone：

Insurance card No. ：

Date：   Time：

Preferred doctor：

Is this your first visit to our hospital?

□ Yes   □ No

Reasons for visit：

Extended Knowledge

Ⅰ. First Aid—Sprained Ankle

Step 1 Determine the severity of the sprain.

Sprains come in three grades. Grade one sprain has slight tearing of the ligaments, and will result in mild tenderness and swelling. Grade two sprain has partial ligament tearing, moderate tenderness and swelling. Grade three sprain is a complete tear of the ligaments, and will have significant swelling and tenderness around the ankle.

1. Grade one sprain usually does not require medical attention. Grade three sprain should almost be seen by a doctor to make sure there is no other damage to the ankle.

2. Home treatment and management for all three grades is the same, but the higher the grade, the longer it will take for the ankle to heal.

Step 2 See your doctor for moderate or severe sprain.

Grade one sprain may not require any medical attention, but grade two or grade three sprain should be seen by a doctor. If your sprain prevents you from comfortably putting weight on your ankle for more than a day, or if you experience severe pain and swelling, make an appointment with a doctor as soon as possible.

Step 3 Rest your ankle until the swelling goes down.

Step 4 Ice your ankle to limit swelling and dull pain.

Apply ice to your ankle even if you plan to go to the doctor. Ice limits swelling and bruising, especially during the first 24 hours of the injury.

Step 5 Compress your ankle with an elastic bandage.

Use a compression bandage, an elastic bandage, or an elastic brace to help manage swelling. Wrap the bandage around the ankle and foot, and secure it with metal fasteners or medical tape. Be

Note

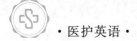

sure to keep the wrap dry.

Step 6 Elevate your ankle above the level of your heart.

Sit back or lie down and use an ottoman to elevate your ankle. Keep your ankle elevated for 2 to 3 hours a day until your ankle stops swelling.

Step 7 Take an over-the-counter pain reliever.

Over-the-counter pain medications such as aspirin and ibuprofen are typically strong enough to help manage the pain and inflammation that goes with a sprained ankle. Use the packaging to help you determine the correct dose, and take it as recommended to manage any pain and swelling.

Ⅱ. Knowledge Links

How to Prepare for a Doctor's Appointment

In western countries, when you get sick, you are supposed to make an appointment with a doctor before visiting. But how to communicate your problems effectively? The following tips may be helpful for you.

1. Create a list of current medications, including the name of the medication, dosage, and how often you take it.

2. Remember your allergies or sensitivities, including medications, foods and body care products.

3. Document your family history. Be prepared to answer many questions about family history. If there are things that are very specific or you think you may forget, make sure to write them down.

4. Bring your medical records. Bring copies of films and test results that were performed since last seeing this doctor.

5. Write down your questions. You may feel stressed at the doctor's office, sometimes it is difficult to remember all the questions you have. To make sure you get the answer, write down questions you concern ahead of time.

6. Bring a family member or friend. Your partner can help you remember what the doctor said during the appointment, they can help ask questions you may not think of, and of course, the extra moral support comes in handy too.

扫码看
答案

Note

Unit 2　Outpatient Service

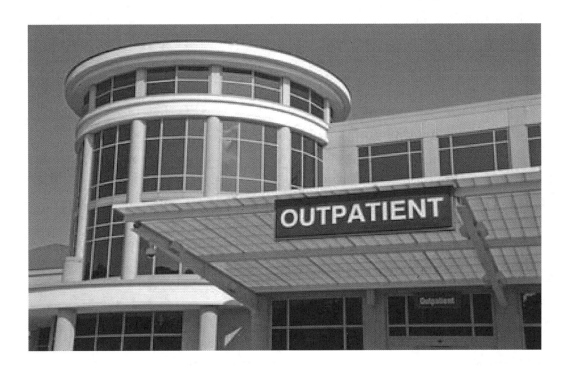

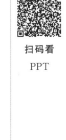

扫码看
PPT

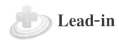 **Lead-in**

Outpatient service refers to medical procedures or tests that can be done in a medical center without an overnight stay. A hospital will usually offer both outpatient service and inpatient service. Outpatient differs from inpatient simply because of that overnight stay.

Outpatient service usually receives the patient with mild minor physical problems, and perhaps some very minor surgeries that does not require an overnight stay. The outpatient doctor gives the patient a primary diagnosis through a complete set of medical means and tests. And if the patient's condition is serious or critical, then he/she is advised to stay in hospital for further examination and treatment. According to the patient's condition, urgent degree and health condition, it can be divided into general outpatient service, healthcare outpatient service and emergency outpatient service.

Thinking & Talking

1. What is the outpatient service?
2. State an outpatient service experience.

Note

Focus Listening

Conversation 1

Directions：*You will hear a conversation between a doctor and a patient. Choose the best answer for each of the following questions.*

1. What's troubling the patient? _____.

A. Stomach   B. Head   C. Tooth

2. Which of the following item is NOT mentioned about the patient's supper in the text? _____.

A. Seafood   B. Candy   C. Roast duck

3. What did the patient get tested? _____.

A. Blood   B. Stool   C. Biopsy

4. When did the patient take the report? _____.

A. Immediately   B. A few days later   C. Wait for a while

5. What's the patient advised to avoid for the next few days? _____.

A. Oily food   B. Fruit and vegetable   C. Fried food

New Words & Expressions

stomach ['stʌmək]	n. 胃，胃口
seafood ['siːfuːd]	n. 海鲜，海产食品
vomit ['vɒmɪt]	v. 呕吐；n. 呕吐物
laboratory ['læbərətɔːrɪ]	n. 实验室，研究室
indigestion [ˌɪndɪ'dʒestʃən]	n. 消化不良，不消化
stool [stuːl]	n. 粪便
biopsy ['baɪˌɒpsɪ]	n. 活组织检查，活组织切片检查

Conversation 2

Directions：*Fill in the blanks according to the conversation between a doctor and a patient.*

（A：Doctor   B：Patient）

A：Good morning. What's troubling you?

B：Good morning, doctor. I think I 1. _____.

A：How long have you been sick?

B：For two days.

A：What symptoms do you have?

B：I have a 2. _____ nose and I ache all over.

A：Do you have a fever?

B：I haven't taken my temperature yet, but I feel 3. _____.

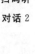

A：Do you have a cough？

B：No，I don't.

A：Do you have 4. _____ ？

B：Yes，my throat feels swollen. It's sore.

A：I want to look at your throat. Open your mouth, please say "ah". It's only a common cold, nothing to worry about. You should rest for a few days and drink more water. I'll write you a certificate for 5. _____ . Here is some Chinese traditional medicine，which is very effective for treating colds. You'll be fine in a few days.

B：Thanks a lot. Bye-bye！

A：Bye！

New Words & Expressions

symptom ['sɪmptəm]	n. 症状，征兆
temperature ['temprətʃə(r)]	n. 温度，体温
swollen ['swəʊlən]	adj. 肿胀的，浮肿的
certificate [sə'tɪfɪkət]	n. 凭证，证书
traditional [trə'dɪʃənəl]	adj. 传统的，惯例的

扫码听
单词

Group Discussion & Role Playing

1. Work in pairs. Suppose a doctor is receiving an outpatient who has been suffering from insomnia for two months. Make a conversation with the following sentences.

• What's troubling you? /What's wrong with you?

• When did you first have the problem? /How long have you been sick?

• Have you taken any medicine?

• Don't worry. / Take it easy.

• Well，there is nothing to be alarmed about.

• I hope you will recover in no time.

2. Work in pairs. Suppose an outpatient is visiting a doctor due to his bad cold. Make a conversation with the instructions below and practice.

Role	Doctor	Outpatient
Step 1	Greet	Greet
Step 2	Inquire about the patient's condition	State the symptoms
Step 3	Make an exam	Active cooperation
Step 4	Comfort the patient and make diagnosis	Show anxiety about the illness
Step 5	Wish a speedy recovery	Express appreciation

Note

扫码听
课文

Intensive Reading

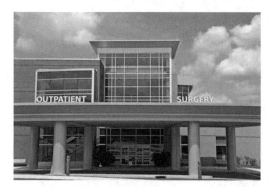

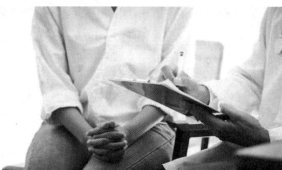

Outpatient Department

Outpatient

An outpatient is someone who goes to a hospital or clinic for the procedure which does not require an overnight stay. The procedure is usually simple and quick, and the patients can often walk in and walk out on their own. Many people have been outpatients at some point in their lives, every time you go to the doctor's office for an exam, a diagnosis for a troubling cold, or a mole removal, you are an outpatient.

Outpatient Surgery

Outpatient surgery refers to those surgeries that usually don't require people to stay overnight in a hospital after they're performed. Most people go home a few hours after having an uncomplicated outpatient surgery. In fact, the number of outpatient surgeries has an increasing trend. There are several reasons why outpatient surgery has become much more popular and safer.

Firstly, surgical techniques have been significantly refined over the last few decades. Some surgeries don't even require huge incisions, which means risk from surgical wounds is extremely minimal. Technology in anesthetic has also improved, making it much easier for people to recover from general anesthetic very quickly and without complication. Studies have also shown that many people recover better at home than in hospital, which can be noisy and may increase the risk of infection. Another driving force behind outpatient surgery expansion is that it lowers cost of medical care. Hospital stays can be expensive and complicated. When they're not necessary, cost reduces significantly.

Outpatient Pharmacy

An outpatient pharmacy is a pharmacy which fills prescriptions for patients affiliated with the pharmacy's parent medical institution, typically a hospital or clinic. Hospitals usually offer outpatient pharmacy services as a convenience to their patients.

There are several advantages for patients who use an outpatient pharmacy as opposed to a regular pharmacy. Firstly, the pharmacy is on the same site where they receive medical treatment, so they do not need to make an extra trip to the pharmacy to pick up prescriptions. Secondly, the pharmacy staff are usually very knowledgeable about the patient's condition. They can quickly catch potential drug conflicts and other issues which may arise. Thirdly, the pharmacy may also offer discounts on

Note

prescriptions.

New Words & Expressions

outpatient [ˈaʊtˌpeɪʃənt]	n. 门诊患者
procedure [prəˈsiːdʒə(r)]	n. 程序,步骤
overnight [ˌəʊvəˈnaɪt]	adj. 晚上的,只供一夜的
diagnosis [ˌdaɪəgˈnəʊsɪs]	n. 诊断
mole [məʊl]	n. 痣,胎块
removal [rɪˈmuːvl]	n. 移除,排除
significantly [sɪgˈnɪfɪkəntlɪ]	adv. 显著地,相当数量地
refine [rɪˈfaɪn]	v. 精炼,改善
incision [ɪnˈsɪʒn]	n. 切口
extremely [ɪkˈstriːmlɪ]	adv. 非常,极端地
minimal [ˈmɪnɪməl]	adj. 最低的,最小限度的
technology [tekˈnɒlədʒɪ]	n. 技术,工艺
anesthetic [ˌænɪsˈθetɪk]	n. 麻醉剂,麻醉药
complication [ˌkɒmplɪˈkeɪʃən]	n. 并发症
infection [ɪnˈfekʃən]	n. 感染,影响
expansion [ɪkˈspænʃən]	n. 膨胀,扩张
pharmacy [ˈfɑːməsɪ]	n. 药房,药学
prescription [prɪˈskrɪpʃən]	n. 药方,处方
affiliate [əˈfɪlɪeɪt]	v. (使)附属,隶属
institution [ˌɪnstɪˈtjuːʃən]	n. 公共机构,制度
convenience [kənˈviːnjəns]	n. 便利,便利的事物
conflict [ˈkɒnflɪkt]	n. 冲突,斗争
discount [ˈdɪskaʊnt]	n. 折扣,贴现率

Exercises

Exercise 1. Choose the best answer for each of the following questions.

1. Which of the subjects are discussed in the text? _____.

A. Outpatient

B. Outpatient surgery

C. Outpatient pharmacy

D. The above all

2. Which of the following patient is an outpatient? _____.

A. A patient who is in the ward after gastrectomy operation

B. A patient who requires surgery quickly due to his acute appendicitis

C. A patient who goes to the doctor's office for his troubling cold

D. A patient who is receiving treatment for cerebroma in the hospital

3. What is the main difference between outpatient surgery and others? _____.

A. Without an overnight stay

B. More convenient

Note

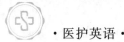

C. More comfortable

D. Cheaper cost

4. According to the text，which is NOT the reason for the popularity of outpatient surgeries? _____.

A. Surgical techniques have been significantly refined

B. Many people recover better at home than they in hospital

C. Outpatient doctor is more professional

D. Outpatient surgery lowers cost of medical care

5. What are the advantages of the outpatient pharmacy，except _____?

A. the pharmacy is on the same site where they receive medical treatment

B. the pharmacy is open during office hours

C. the pharmacy may also offer discounts on prescriptions

D. the pharmacy staff is usually knowledgeable about the patient's condition

Exercise 2. Fill in the blanks with the words given below, changing the form if necessary.

prescribe　　　procedure　　　discount　　　infect

incision　　　pharmacy　　　expansion　　　convenient

1. Hospitals usually offer all kinds of _____ for their patients.

2. The doctor may give you a _____ for some medicine to relieve the symptom.

3. Making an _____ in the eye and removing the lens.

4. I work at a _____ just around the corner from here.

5. My doctor seems to think that this _____ will eventually go away.

Exercise 3. Translate the following Chinese sentences into English.

1. 由于妈妈的细心照顾,海蒂很快就从重感冒中恢复过来。

2. 他们学会了如何诊断类似感冒的普通疾病。

3. 门诊部是隶属于医院的一个综合医疗机构。

4. 患者治疗后更乐意回家而不是住院。

5. 南希需要通过手术来移除发炎的手指头。

Learning More

Ⅰ. Affixes & Roots of Medical Terms

Affixes & Roots	Chinese	More Words
-patient	患者	outpatient 门诊患者；inpatient 住院患者
-itis	炎症	appendicitis 阑尾炎；tonsillitis 扁桃体炎
-tomy	切开术,切除术	gastrectomy 胃切除术；anatomy 解剖学
-ache	疼痛	stomachache 胃痛；headache 头痛
gastr(o)-	胃,胃的	gastroscope 胃镜；gastrocamera 胃内照相机
cerebr(o)-	脑,脑的	cerebroma 脑瘤；cerebroscope 脑镜
rhin-	鼻,鼻的	rhinobyon 鼻塞；rhinitis 鼻炎
auto-	自动的	automated 自动化的；autoimmune 自身免疫的

Affixes & Roots	Chinese	More Words
cardio-	心，心的	cardiopulmonary 心肺的；cardiovascular 心血管的

Match the English expressions with the right Chinese phrases.

1. inpatient   A. 胃内照相机

2. cardiopulmonary   B. 鼻塞

3. autoimmune   C. 住院患者

4. gastrocamera   D. 解剖学

5. anatomy   E. 心肺的

6. appendicitis   F. 脑瘤

7. cerebroma   G. 头痛

8. rhinobyon   H. 阑尾炎

9. headache   I. 鼻炎

10. rhinitis   J. 自身免疫的

Ⅱ. Vocabulary Expansion

Match the Chinese phrases with the right English expressions.

A. complication	B. mole removal	C. outpatient surgery
D. overnight	E. general anesthesia	F. surgical technique
G. drug conflicts	H. outpatient	I. outpatient pharmacy
J. medical institution	K. regular pharmacy	L. treatment

1. (　　)普通药店　　　　(　　)门诊手术

2. (　　)治疗　　　　　　(　　)门诊患者

3. (　　)并发症　　　　　(　　)全身麻醉

4. (　　)门诊药房　　　　(　　)药物冲突

5. (　　)手术技术　　　　(　　)医疗机构

Practical Writing

Outpatient Medical Record（门诊病历）

　　门诊病历是门诊患者过去和现在的健康状况的记录，为医生诊断提供有用的信息。其主要包含以下内容：个人信息、过敏史、主诉、病史、诊断、签名等。

Sample

Outpatient Medical Record

Date：May 2, 2019		Department：ENT（ear, nose and throat）
Name：Nancy Joyce	**Age**：39	**Gender**：female

Note

续表

Occupation：teacher	Marital status：married	Tel. ：138××××××××

Address：Room 301，Building No. 1，Simingyuan Garden，Siming Road，Siming District，Xiamen City

Allergies：no known drug allergy

Chief complaint：sore throat and fever

History of present illness：
1. Suffering a mild sore throat and pharynx dry for the last six months.
2. Having a feeling of headache and tiredness.
3. There is no difficulty in opening the mouth and breathing.

Physical examination：
Temp：38 ℃
The oral mucosa is congested and the tonsils are swollen.

Diagnosis：acute tonsillitis

Signature：Dr. Li Bo

Exercise

Please write an outpatient medical record according to the information given below.

【Heidi，女，学生，10 岁，2016 年随父母移居中国厦门，现住在厦门市思明区思明路思明苑 1 栋 301，联系电话为 138××××××××。2019 年 10 月 12 日开始鼻塞，咳嗽，两天后病情加重，在妈妈陪伴下来医院就诊。患者自述两天前因为受凉出现鼻塞，咳嗽，今天开始发烧，无恶心呕吐和呼吸困难等症状，无药物过敏史。查体：体温 38.5 ℃，心率 95 次/分，双肺无湿啰音。布莱克医生的诊断：急性上呼吸道感染。】

Outpatient Medical Record

Date：		Department：	
Name：	Age：		Sex：
Occupation：	Marital status：		Tel. ：
Address：			
Allergies：			
Chief complaint：			
History of present illness：			
Physical examination：			
Diagnosis：			
Signature：			

Extended Knowledge

I. First Aid—Heart Attack

Step 1 Call emergency service.

Don't ignore or attempt to tough out the symptoms of a heart attack. If you don't have access to emergency medical services, have a neighbor or a friend drive you to the nearest hospital. Drive yourself only as a last resort, and realize that it places you and others at risk when you drive under the circumstance.

Step 2 Chew and swallow an aspirin.

Unless you are allergic to aspirin or have been told by your doctor never to take aspirin.

Step 3 Take nitroglycerin.

If you think you're having a heart attack and your doctor has previously prescribed nitroglycerin for you, take it as directed. Don't take anyone else's nitroglycerin, because that could put you in more danger.

Step 4 Begin CPR if the person is unconscious.

If you're with a person who is unconscious, tell the 120 dispatcher or another emergency medical specialist. You may be advised to begin cardiopulmonary resuscitation (CPR). If you haven't received CPR training, doctors recommend performing only chest compressions (about 100 to 120 compressions a minute). The dispatcher can instruct you in the proper procedures until help arrives.

Step 5 Using AED.

If an automated external defibrillator (AED) is immediately available and the person is unconscious, follow the device instructions for using it.

II. Knowledge Links

Cardiopulmonary Resuscitation (CPR)

Cardiopulmonary resuscitation (CPR) is a lifesaving technique useful in many emergencies, including a heart attack or near drowning, in which someone's breathing or heartbeat has stopped.

Here is a step-by-step guide for the new CPR.

Step 1 Call emergency services or ask someone else to do so.

Step 2 Keep the victim on his or her back.

Try to get the person to respond, if he doesn't, roll the person on his or her back while trying to support his or her head and neck.

Step 3 Start chest compressions.

Place the heel of your hand on the center of the victim's chest. Put your other hand on top of the first with your fingers interlaced. Press down the chest at least 2 inches in adults or children and 1.5 inches in infants. One hundred times a minute or even a little faster is optimal.

Step 4 Open the airway.

If you've been trained in CPR, you can now open the airway with a head tilt and chin lift.

Note

17

Step 5 Breathe for the victim.

Pinch closed the nose of the victim. Take a normal breath，cover the victim's mouth with yours to create an airtight seal，then give two，one-second breaths as you watch for the chest to rise.

Continue with compressions and breaths（30 compressions，two breaths）until help arrives.

Unit 3   Pharmacy

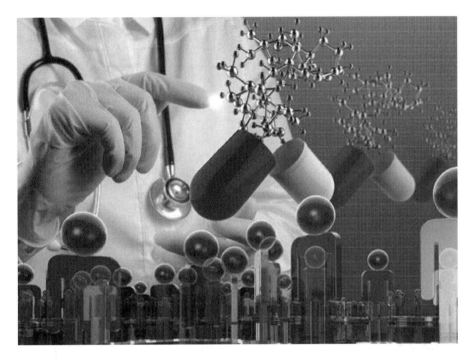

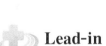 **Lead-in**

Hospitals usually offer outpatient pharmacy services as a convenience to their patients. As with other types of pharmacies, an outpatient pharmacy can usually handle written prescriptions as well as prescriptions which are phoned in. Due to the need to compound complex drugs in a hospital facility, these pharmacies may also be able to offer specialty drugs and preparations to their patients.

In addition to an outpatient pharmacy, hospitals also have an inpatient pharmacy, which specifically fills prescriptions for people who are hospitalized. The inpatient pharmacy is often in a different area of the hospital from the outpatient one, with doctors picking up prescriptions for their patients. This pharmacy also synchronizes its records with the outpatient pharmacy to ensure that the patient's data is always up to date.

Thinking & Talking

1. Please list the route of administration that you know.
2. What responsibilities would you take if you were a pharmacist or a nurse?

Note

19

Focus Listening

Conversation 1

扫码听
对话 1

Directions：*You will hear a conversation between <u>Ms．Zheng</u> and <u>a chemist</u>．They are in a Chinese medicinal herbs store．Listen to the conversation and decide whether the following statements are true（T）or false（F）．*

（　　）1. Before decoction，the patient needs to soak the herbs.

（　　）2. Simmer for twenty minutes after it begins to boil.

（　　）3. The patient should not let any of the leaves go into the cup.

（　　）4. The patient can also use a steel pan to decoct Chinese herbs.

（　　）5. One dose of herbal medicine can be used twice.

New Words & Expressions

扫码听
单词

herbal ['hɜːbəl]   adj. 草药的；n. 草本植物志

decoction [dɪ'kɒkʃən]   n. 煎煮，煎熬的药

soak [səʊk]   v. 浸泡，渗透

boil [bɔɪl]   v. 煮沸；n. 沸点

simmer ['sɪmə(r)]   v. 炖，煨

earthenware ['ɜːθənweə(r)]   adj. 陶制的；n. 陶器

dose [dəʊs]   n. 剂量；v. 服药

Conversation 2

扫码听
对话 2

Directions：*You will hear a conversation between <u>Chen Hong</u> and <u>a chemist</u>．Chen Hong has a bad cold and now she is in a pharmacy．Listen carefully and fill in the blanks according to the conversation．*

（A：Chemist　B：Chen Hong）

A：Good morning. May I help you?

B：Good morning. I have a 1._____cold. Could you sell me some antibiotic medicine?

A：Do you have a prescription?

B：No，I haven't gone to see a doctor.

A：Sorry, sir. I cannot sell it to you. You must first get a doctor's prescription, and then I can fill it for you. But I can 2._____ some OTC medicine to 3._____ the symptoms of cold.

B：I see. Could you suggest something I can take to relieve the headache?

A：We have a number of 4._____. They are all very good. How about this brand?

B：All right. How do I take this medicine?

A：Take one tablet whenever you feel pain，but do not take more than 5._____.

B：Thank you very much.

A：You're welcome. I hope you will 6._____ soon.

扫码听
单词

New Words & Expressions

antibiotic [ˌæntɪbaɪˈɒtɪk]	adj. 抗菌的;n. 抗生素
OTC (over-the-counter) medicine	非处方药
relieve [rɪˈliːv]	v. 减轻,解除
brand [brænd]	n. 品牌,商标
tablet [ˈtæblət]	n. 药片

Group Discussion & Role Playing

1. Discuss with your partner. Change the patient types or demands and redesign the conversation.

2. Display the conversation you've made.

3. After one group finishes the performance, others make comments.

Intensive Reading

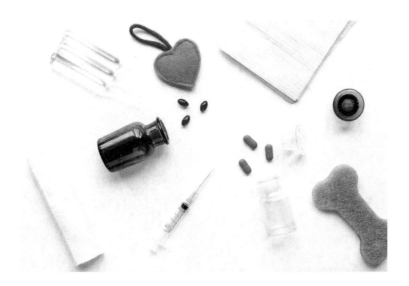

扫码听
课文

How to Administer Medication Correctly

Medication plays an important role in the prevention, diagnosis and treatment of diseases. In order to promote the health of patients, medical staff must adopt the correct administration methods and routes to achieve appropriate treatment effect.

1. Check the "Five Rights" before administering medication.

At first, you must check the "Five Rights". The "Five Rights" refers to the right patient, the right drug, the right dose, the right route and the right time and frequency. For example, along with the patient's name, ask for his date of birth to make sure the prescription matches the patient.

2. Ask the patient about allergies and reactions to medications before any new medication is

Note

administered.

3. Avoid abbreviations, which can be easily misinterpreted when documenting medication allergies.

4. Pay close attention to the patient's critical diagnose, smoking, alcohol, and substance used which can affect not only the selection of medication but also dose and frequency, especially the patients with kidney, liver, psychiatric diseases, diabetes mellitus and pregnant women.

5. Note the patient's current medication regimen and update the list at each doctor's visit. This should be documented in the same location on his chart so it's easy to locate. Not only should you document the dose and frequency of prescribed medications, but also any OTC (over-the-counter), herbs or supplements.

6. Learn and differentiate drug names that are similar. Most of the drugs that sound similar but different uses. For instance, the drug Celebrex is commonly used to treat arthritis while the similarly named Cerebyx is used to treat seizures.

7. Store "high alert" or similar-sounding drugs in separate areas so they won't be easily confused. Make sure the drug storage area is well organized. Go through your medication storage area at least quarterly. Discard any expired medication and make sure medication labels are easy to read and facing forward on the shelf.

扫码听
单词

New Words & Expressions

administer [əd'mɪnɪstə(r)]	v. 给予,管理
administration [əd,mɪnɪ'streɪʃən]	n.（药物的）施用
appropriate [ə'prəʊprɪət]	adj. 适当的；v. 占用
abbreviation [ə,briːvɪ'eɪʃən]	n. 缩写
misinterpret [,mɪsɪn'tɜːprɪt]	v. 误解,曲解
substance ['sʌbstəns]	n. 物质,实质
psychiatric [,saɪkɪ'ætrɪk]	adj. 精神病学的,精神病治疗的
mellitus ['melɪtəs]	n. 糖尿病
regimen ['redʒɪmən]	n. 方案,生活规则
supplement ['sʌplɪmənt]	n. 补品,增补（物）
differentiate [,dɪfə'renʃɪeɪt]	v. 区分,区别
arthritis [ɑː'θraɪtɪs]	n. 关节炎
seizure ['siːʒə(r)]	n.（疾病）发作
separate ['seprət]	adj. 分开的；v. 使分离
storage ['stɔːrɪdʒ]	n. 存储,仓库
quarterly ['kwɔːtəlɪ]	adv. 按季度地
discard [dɪ'skɑːd]	v. 丢弃,抛弃
expire [ɪk'spaɪə(r)]	v. 到期,终止
label ['leɪbəl]	n. 标签,商标

Exercises

Exercise 1. Decide whether the following statements are true (T) or false (F) according to the text.

Note

(   ) 1. The "Five Rights" refers to the right drug, the right patient, the right dose, the right route and the right time and frequency.

( ) 2. You are allowed to use abbreviations when documenting medication allergies.

( ) 3. You just need to record the prescribed medications and OTC medicine.

( ) 4. Cerebyx is commonly used to treat arthritis.

( ) 5. Check your medication storage area at least every three months.

Exercise 2. Fill in the blanks with the words given below, changing the form if necessary.

discard   storage   supplement   substance

dose   label   misinterpret   update

1. Madame Curie discovered the radioactive _____ of radium and polonium in 1988.

2. Abbreviations can be easily _____.

3. The patient's critical diagnoses can affect not only the selection of medication but also _____ and frequency.

4. Note the patient's current medication regimen and _____ the list at each doctor's visit.

5. Make sure the drug _____ area is well organized.

Exercise 3. Translate the following Chinese sentences into English.

1. 为了促进患者的健康,医护人员必须采用正确的给药方法和途径才能达到应有的治疗效果。

2. 在询问患者姓名的同时,询问他的出生日期,以确保处方与患者匹配。

3. 在服用任何新药之前,请询问患者对药物的过敏史和反应情况。

4. 患者在这些问题上的病史有助于药物治疗决策,包括剂量和频次。

5. 丢弃所有过期的药物,并确保药物标签易于阅读并面向货架。

Learning More

I. Affixes & Roots of Medical Terms

Affixes & Roots	Chinese	More Words
ante-	在……之前	antecibum 饭前;antenatal 产前的
anti-	与……相反,反对	antitoxin 抗毒素;antibiotic 抗生素
cef-	头孢	ceftazidime 头孢他啶;cefalexin 头孢氨苄
intra-	在……内	intravenous 静脉内;intramuscular 肌肉内
-cillin	青霉素类抗生素	penicillin 青霉素

Match the English expressions with the right Chinese phrases.

1. antibody   A. 羧苄青霉素

2. carbenicillin   B. 头孢噻肟

3. intracellular   C. 抗病毒素

4. antecedent   D. 抗体

5. cefotaxime   E. 细胞内的

6. antivirus   F. 前情,祖先

Note

Ⅱ. Vocabulary Expansion

Match the Chinese phrases with the right English expressions.

A. Rx.	B. t. i. d.	C. p. r. n.
D. p. c.	E. I. V.	F. sig.
G. h. s.	H. Caps.	I. tab.
J. q. i. d.	K. p. o.	L. a. c.

1. (　　)用法用量　　　　(　　)按情酌定
2. (　　)静脉注射　　　　(　　)每日三次
3. (　　)睡前　　　　　　(　　)饭前
4. (　　)片剂　　　　　　(　　)处方
5. (　　)胶囊　　　　　　(　　)口服

Practical Writing

Prescription(处方)

处方应该包含以下内容。
1. 处方的标题和开具日期。
2. 患者的基本信息,如姓名、性别、年龄。
3. 药品剂量、规格、用法用量。
4. 医生签字。

Sample

Prescription
Name：Wang Yuan　　　**Age**：35　　　**Date**：Aug. 8，2020
Address：No. 105，Guangan Road，Xuanwu District，Beijing
Rx.：Throat lozenge 100 mg/tab.
Sig.：Six tabs. daily.
Disp.：50 tabs.
Name of doctor：Wang Wei
Signature：*Wang Wei*

Exercise

Fill in the blanks of a description according to the information.

【陈东,40 岁,家住北京市海淀区延安路 20 号。他喉咙痛并发烧,于 2019 年 7 月 12 日去医院就诊。吴林医生诊断为重感冒。处方用药为:①阿司匹林,0.5 克×8 片,每次 1 片,每天 3 次,饭后服用。②润喉片 100 毫克×30 片,每 4 小时 1 次,每次 1 片,每天 6 次。】

Prescription

Name：_____ Age：_____ Date：_____

Address：_____

Rx. : _____

Sig. : _____

Disp. : _____

Name of doctor：_____

Signature：_____

Extended Knowledge

I . First Aid—Animal Bites Treatment

Step 1 Stop bleeding.

Apply direct pressure until bleeding stops.

Step 2 Clean and protect.

1. For a wound or superficial scratch from an animal bite, gently clean with soap and warm water. Rinse for several minutes after cleaning.

2. Apply antibiotic cream to reduce risk of infection, and cover with a sterile bandage.

Step 3 Get help.

1. Get medical help immediately for any animal bite that is more than a superficial scratch or if the animal was a wild animal or stray, regardless of the severity of the injury.

2. If the animal's owner is available, find out if the animal's rabies shots are up-to-date. Give this information to your health care provider.

3. If the animal was a stray or wild animal, call the local health department or animal control immediately.

Step 4 Find the health care provider for more help.

Call for the emergency services if：

1. Bleeding can't be stopped after 10 minutes of firm and steady pressure.

2. Bleeding is severe or blood spurts from the wound.

II . Knowledge Links

The Intravenous Injection

The intravenous injection is a means of delivering additional medication through an intravenous line, administered all at once, over a period of a minute or two. This contrasts with I. V. drip techniques where medicine is slowly delivered from an I. V. bag. An I. V. push has the advantage of being able to give extra medicine as needed, without having to inject the patient elsewhere, and it can rapidly get this medicine into the body since it's injected directly into the bloodstream. This technique also comes with noted cautions, since not all medicines can be delivered this way and some may cause extreme irritation or toxically high blood levels of a medicine, if they are given too quickly.

扫码看
答案

Note

Unit 4　Hospital Admission and Discharge

扫码看
PPT

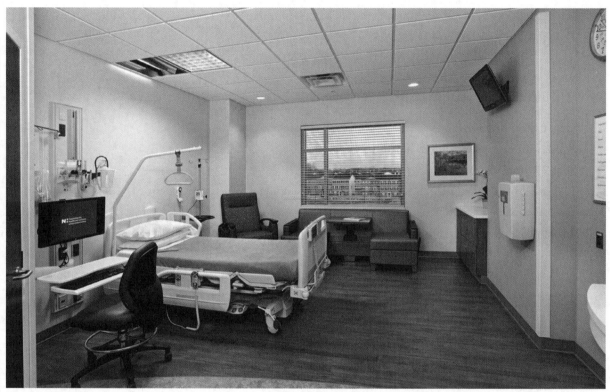

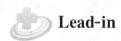

Lead-in

The admission procedure includes emergency admission and pre-arranged admission. The nurses perform the admission procedure, for example, filling in an admission card, introducing environment and regulations of the ward, gathering the patient's information and so on. Usually, registration is the first step for seeing a doctor in hospital.

Thinking & Talking

1. Do you know the admission procedure? Can you draw an admission flow chart?

2. What services may discharge plan involve?

Note

Focus Listening

Conversation 1

Directions：*Mr. Smith is going to be admitted to the hospital. Now he is talking with the nurse about something important for admission. Listen carefully and decide whether the following statements are true (T) or false (F).*

(　　) 1. The nurse will bring the patient to the ward.

(　　) 2. The patient will stay in the hospital for three days.

(　　) 3. The hospital cannot provide daily necessities for the patient.

(　　) 4. There are some shops on the fourth floor.

扫码听
对话 1

New Words & Expressions

admission [əd'mɪʃən]	n. 承认,入院
ward [wɔːd]	n. 病房,监视
elevator ['elɪveɪtə(r)]	n. 电梯,升降机
walk over	走过去
mount up	增加

扫码听
单词

Conversation 2

Directions：*Mrs. Wang is in the ward. Now a nurse is introducing the surrounding of the ward to her. Fill in the blanks according to the conversation between the nurse and Mrs. Wang.*

1. Why does Mrs. Wang say "nice meeting you"?

　　It's a way of ＿＿＿＿.

2. When can Mrs. Wang use the tub and shower room?

　　From ＿＿＿＿ in the morning to ＿＿＿＿ in the evening.

3. What will happen when Mrs. Wang presses the call button?

　　The nurse will ＿＿＿＿.

4. What should Mrs. Wang keep in her bedside table?

　　Small things, such as ＿＿＿＿ and ＿＿＿＿.

扫码听
对话 2

New Words & Expressions

tub [tʌb]	n. 浴盆,桶
occupied ['ɒkjupaɪd]	adj. 已占用的
nightgown ['naɪtgaʊn]	n. 睡衣
call button	呼叫按钮
toilet articles	盥洗用品

扫码听
单词

Note

扫码听
课文

Group Discussion & Role Playing

1. Discuss with your partner. Change the patient types or demands and redesign the conversation.
2. Display the conversation you've made.
3. After one group finishes the performance, others make comments.

Intensive Reading

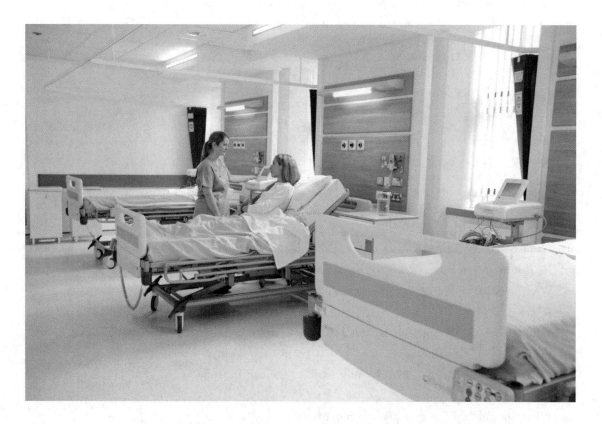

Admission to the Hospital

In order to evaluate the patient's clinical condition and nursing needs, patients can't avoid to perform the admission procedure which also serves as a method to collect data.

Pre-admission and Registration

When the patients are coming for admission, please check the following items.

1. The attending doctor will give the patient an admission card or notice. Because inpatient admission to the hospital is permissible only upon the recommendation of a doctor.

2. Admission form which includes personal data, medical history, reasons for admission, action to be taken and others is necessary.

3. The patient had better bring his/her ID card, national health insurance IC card and related certificates.

Note

4. The patient's previous medical records, test results, X-rays and a list of the medications which the patient is presently taking should be ready.

5. The patient should pay the deposit in advance.

About the Admission Procedure

1. When the admission office confirms when the patients will hospitalize, a nurse will call to inform the specific date. The patient or his/her relative should deal with the inpatient procedures in the informed time. Otherwise, the beds would not be reserved.

2. The underclothing and daily necessities should be prepared by the patient himself/herself. The patient should keep in mind: do not bring valuables when hospitalized.

3. Arrival at the Hospital

On the admission day, the patient should bring all of the items mentioned above, hand them in at the admission office and sign a hospitalization agreement. After that, the patient will be taken to the respective ward.

4. Arrival at the Ward

After arriving at the ward, the hospital will provide a ward orientation and instant medical care. Once the patient reaches the ward, he/she will be escorted to the allocated bed and a ward team member will familiarize the patient with the surroundings.

In order to get concise medical and social history, the nurse will come to ask a series of questions. To help the anesthetist calculate the necessary dose of medication, the nurse will measure the patient's weight and height. To act as a baseline measurement prior to surgery, the nurse will also take the patient's BP (blood pressure), HR (heart rate), oxygen saturation level and temperature.

New Words & Expressions

inpatient [ˈɪnpeɪʃənt]	n. 住院患者
presently [ˈprezntlɪ]	adv. 现在
inform [ɪnˈfɔːm]	v. 通知
reserve [rɪˈzɜːv]	v. 留出，保留
familiarize [fəˈmɪljəraɪz]	v. 使熟悉
anesthetist [æˈniːsθətɪst]	n. 麻醉师
calculate [ˈkælkjʊleɪt]	v. 计算
saturation [ˌsætʃəˈreɪʃən]	n. 饱和
clinical condition	临床状况
pay the deposit	支付押金
escort to	护送
baseline measurement	基准测量

扫码听
单词

Exercises

Exercise 1. Read the passage and decide whether the following statements are true (T) or false (F).

( ) 1. Nurses will take the patient's baseline-functions like heart rate, temperature and blood pressure.

( ) 2. When arriving at the hospital, a nurse or other hospital staff will begin with the admission procedure by asking questions about the patient's medical history.

( ) 3. The patient will receive a letter about the proposal date of admission.

Note

(　) 4. When arriving at the ward, the nurse will lead the patient to the allocated bed.

(　) 5. In order to give the patient the accurate amount of anesthetic, the anesthetist will have the patient's medical information, such as age, height and weight.

Exercise 2. Fill in the blanks with the words given below, changing the form if necessary.

| give | include | suggest | arrive |
| hospital | sign | check | permissible |

1. The admission card is _____ by the patient's attending doctor.

2. After the patient _____ at the ward, a ward orientation and immediate medical care will be provided.

3. It is _____ that the deposit in accordance with the schedule of charges be paid in advance.

4. Please do not bring precious articles when _____.

5. The patients are required to _____ a hospitalization agreement and then will be taken to the respective ward.

Exercise 3. Arrange the following steps in a proper sequence based on the admission procedure.

A. Scheduling of hospitalization

B. Notification of hospitalization

C. Pre-admission and registration

D. Admission

The correct order of admission procedure is _____.

Exercise 4. Translate the following Chinese sentences into English.

1. 患者不可避免地要办理入院手续，这也是收集资料的一种方法。

2. 医疗助理向患者介绍医院的环境、护理体系以及其在体系中的角色。

3. 提供包含个人资料、病史、入院原因和将采取的治疗措施等内容的入院表格也是必要的。

4. 患者需要自己准备内衣和日常生活用品。

5. 为了获得患者的简明医疗史和社交史，护士将会来问患者一系列问题。

Learning More

Ⅰ. Affixes & Roots of Medical Terms

Affixes & Roots	Chinese	More Words
-itis	炎症	gastroenteritis 肠胃炎；hepatitis 肝炎
re-	再，重新，重复	rehydration 复水，再水化；relapse 复发
dis-	否定，去除，反面	discharge 释放，出院；disorder 使失调
naus-	船	nausea 作呕，晕船
ap-(ad-)	加强，增强	appetite 食欲

Match the English expressions with the right Chinese phrases.

1. appetite   A. 作呕，晕船

2. discharge   B. 食欲

3. nausea   C. 释放，出院

4. gastroenteritis   D. 肠胃炎

5. rehydration   E. 复发

6. relapse   F. 复水,再水化

Ⅱ. Vocabulary Expansion

Match the Chinese phrases with the right English expressions.

A. notification of hospitalization	B. sign a hospitalization agreement	C. admission card/notice
D. the bed allotment	E. oxygen saturation level	F. medical history
G. a baseline measurement	H. the unit's environment	I. record vital signs
J. oral or nasal suctioning	K. nasogastric feed	L. maintain the airway open

1. (   )保持气道开放   (   )安排病床

2. (   )基准测量   (   )在住院协议上签字

3. (   )病房环境   (   )病历

4. (   )入院卡或入院通知   (   )血氧饱和度

5. (   )住院通知   (   )鼻饲

Practical Writing

Discharge Summary(出院小结)

出院小结是患者在住院期间的诊断、诊疗经过以及出院指导的简要说明。其内容主要包含以下几个方面。

1. 入院、出院日期,住院天数。

2. 入院时病情摘要及入院诊断。住院期间的病情变化及诊疗经过。

3. 出院时情况,包括出院时存在的症状、体征、疾病的恢复程度、后遗症等。

4. 出院诊断。

5. 出院指导,包括注意事项和建议,需继续服用的药物名称、数量、剂量、用法。

6. 出院记录,在出院后 24 小时内完成。

Sample

Patient：John	Gender：male	Age：15
HOD (hospital day)	7 days	
DOA (date of admission)	Oct. 10, 2019	
Attending physician	Chen Feng	
Conditions on admission	vomiting	
AD (admitting diagnosis)	acute gastroenteritis	
Hospital course	The patient was admitted and placed on fluid rehydration and mineral supplement.	

Note

31

续表

DOD（date of discharge）	Oct. 17，2019
Conditions on discharge	1. The patient becomes better. 2. There is a remission of nausea and vomiting. 3. The patient is in a stable condition. 4. The patient can discharge from the hospital duly.
DD（discharge diagnosis）	acute gastroenteritis
Prognosis	Excellent. No medications needed after discharge. But in order to prevent the relapse（复发）of acute gastroenteritis, the patient had better take some bland diet.

The patient is to follow up with Dr. Chen in one week.

Signature：*Dr. Chen*

Date：Oct. 17，2019

Exercise

Read the information below and fill in the discharge summary.

The patient who called Wang Li is 18 years old. She was admitted because of dizziness，headache and blurred vision on Oct. 7，2019. At the beginning，she was diagnosed as hypertension and placed on anti-hypertensive drugs by attending physician Dr. Lin. Sixteen days later，the patient became better，showing general state of health，and the symptom of dizziness，headache and blurred vision had disappeared. The patient was discharged in stable condition. Finally，she was diagnosed as hypertension. The patient should follow up with Dr. Lin in one week.

Patient：_____	Gender：_____	Age：_____
HOD（hospital day）	_____	
DOA（date of admission）	_____	
Attending physician	_____	
Conditions on admission	_____	
AD（admitting diagnosis）	_____	
Hospital course	_____	
DOD（date of discharge）	_____	
Conditions on discharge	_____	
DD（discharge diagnosis）	_____	
Prognosis	_____	

The patient is to follow up with Dr. Lin in one week.

Signature：_____

Date：Oct. 23，2019

Extended Knowledge

Ⅰ. First Aid—Near Drowning: On-site First Aid Steps

Step 1 Rescued the downing person from the water.

To improve the respiratory function of drowning people and minimize the time of hypoxia, the drowning person should be quickly rescued from the water.

Step 2 Keep the airway open.

Keep the airway open, and immediately pry the open cavity to clear the mud, weeds, and vomit in the mouth and nose, and remove them with dentures to prevent falling into the airway. Loose the tight underwear, belts and others to ensure smooth breathing.

Step 3 Quickly drain the water in the lungs and stomach.

The following methods can be used to quickly drain the water in the respiratory tract and stomach of the drowning person.

1. Knee top method. The rescuer takes a half-squat position, kneels on one leg, flexes the other leg, and places the drowning people's abdomen on the rescuer's thigh. Keep the drowning people's head drooping, and press his back to make the water in the respiratory pour out.

2. Shoulder top method. The rescuer embraces the drowning people's legs, puts his abdomen on the shoulder of the rescuer, and drowns the drowning people's head and chest, which is conducive to the drainage of water.

3. Abdomen holding method. The rescuer hugs the drowning people's waist and abdomen with both hands from the back, so that the drowning people's back is on the top. And his head and abdomen should sag to make the accumulated water pour out. Note that the pouring time should not be too long.

Step 4 Performed cardiopulmonary resuscitation.

If the drowning person has breathing or heart stopped, he/she should immediately be performed cardiopulmonary resuscitation.

Step 5 Quickly send drowning person to hospital for treatment.

Ⅱ. Knowledge Links

What is an ICU?

An intensive care unit (ICU) is a special facility within a hospital that is dedicated to treating patients who are critically ill. The patients may be experiencing multiple organ failure, respiratory arrest, or other serious problems that require intensive monitoring. The staff are specially trained to administer critical care, and there are sometimes several staffers assigned to each patient to ensure that patients get the care they need.

Intensive care medicine focuses on the major systems of the body, including the cardiovascular system, the gastrointestinal tract, the central nervous system, and the respiratory tract. Providers try to keep these important bodily systems running smoothly so that the patient remains stable. As the patient's underlying condition is treated, smoothly running bodily systems will greatly improve the patient's prognosis. In a very unstable patient, ICU care may require constant adjustment of medications and treatment programs, along with a very focused and dedicated staff.

扫码看
答案

Note

33

Unit 5　Medical Imaging

扫码看
PPT

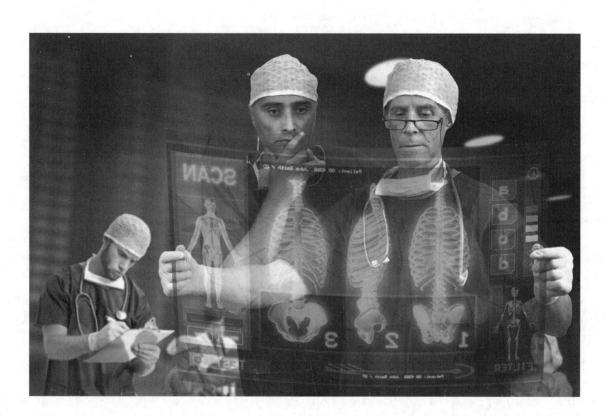

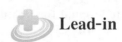 **Lead-in**

Medical imaging is a discipline within the medical field which involves the use of technology to take images of the inside of the human body. These images are used in diagnostics, as teaching tools, and in routine healthcare for a variety of conditions. Medical imaging is sometimes referred to as diagnostic imaging, because it is frequently used to help doctors arrive at a diagnosis, and there are a number of different types of technology used in imaging.

The goal of imaging is to provide a picture of the inside of the body in a way that is as non-invasive as possible. An imaging study can be used to identify unusual things inside the body, such as broken bones, tumors, leaking blood vessels, etc. One of the most famous types of diagnostic imaging is the X-ray, which uses radiation to take a static image of a specific area of the body.

Thinking & Talking

1. Have you ever had the experience of being taken a medical image?
2. What other types of diagnostic imaging do you know?

Note

Focus Listening

Conversation 1

Directions: *You will hear a conversation between* <u>*Doctor Murray*</u> *and* <u>*Mark*</u>*. Doctor Murray is doing a physical test for Mark. Listen carefully and decide whether the following statements are true (T) or false (F).*

(　　) 1. The first test of Mark is his stomach function test.

(　　) 2. Mark can understand the first test he was taken at the very beginning.

(　　) 3. The thyroid gland produces a chemical messenger called hormone.

(　　) 4. Mark has diabetes before his treatment.

(　　) 5. Carbohydrate makes your blood sugar go down, while insulin and exercise keep your blood sugar levels up.

扫码听
对话 1

New Words & Expressions

thyroid [ˈθaɪrɔɪd]	n. 甲状腺
function [ˈfʌŋkʃən]	n. 功能
accelerator [əkˈseləreɪtə(r)]	n. 催化剂
chemical [ˈkemɪkəl]	n. 化学制品
thyroxin [θaɪˈrɔksɪn]	n. 甲状腺素
blood sugar	血糖
carbohydrate [ˌkɑːbəʊˈhaɪdreɪt]	n. 碳水化合物,糖类
insulin [ˈɪnsjʊlɪn]	n. 胰岛素
balance [ˈbæləns]	v. 平衡

扫码听
单词

Conversation 2

Directions: *Robert is calling the hospital in California where Mrs. Marshall received treatment ten days ago. Listen and fill in the blanks in his notes.*

PMH (previous medical history):

CC (chief complaint): 1. _____ pain.

On admission:

ECG(electrocardiogram): ST segment and T wave 2. _____.

Diagnosis: Myocardial 3. _____. Rx: Morphine 2 mg I. V., 4. _____, and put her under 5. _____.

After 6/24: She responded very well and after six hours, her T waves were looking much better.

扫码听
对话 2

New Words & Expressions

stroke [strəʊk]	n. 中风
myocardial [ˌmaɪəʊˈkɑːdɪəl]	adj. 心肌的

扫码听
单词

Note

infarction [ɪnˈfɑːkʃən]	n. 梗塞
intravenous [ˌɪntrəˈviːnəs]	adj. 静脉内的
electrocardiogram [ɪˌlektrəʊˈkɑːdɪəʊɡræm]	n. 心电图
ST segment [ˈseɡmənt]	ST 段（心电图）
abnormality [ˌæbnɔːˈmælətɪ]	n. 异常，畸形
morphine [ˈmɔːfiːn]	n. 吗啡
aspirin [ˈæsprɪn]	n. 阿司匹林
heparin [ˈhepərɪn]	n. 肝素

Group Discussion & Role Playing

1. Discuss with your partner. Change the role of the patient and the doctor and redesign the conversation.

2. Display the conversation you've made.

3. After one group finishes the performance, others make comments.

Intensive Reading

扫码听
课文

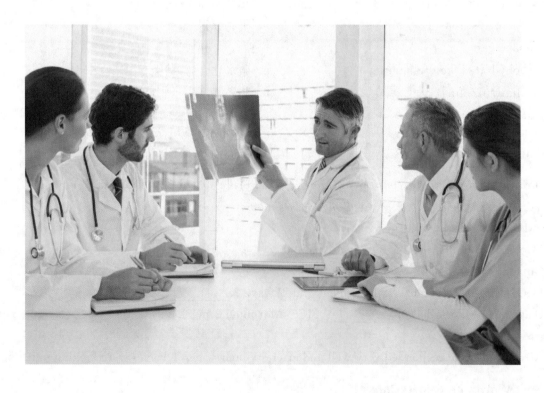

Radiology

Radiology is the medical specialty concerned with the study of X-rays. X-rays are invisible waves of energy which are produced by an energy source (X-ray machine or Cathode tube). Several

Note

characteristics of X-rays are useful to physicians in the diagnosis and treatment of diseases.

Some of these characteristics are：

1. Ability to cause exposure of a photographic plate. If a photographic plate is placed in front of a beam of X-rays, the X-rays, travelling unimpededly through the air, will expose the silver coating of the plate and cause it to blacken.

2. Ability to penetrate different substances to varying degrees. X-rays pass through the different types of substances in the human body with varying ease.

If the X-rays are absorbed (stopped) by the body substance (e. g. calcium in bones), they do not reach the photographic plate held behind the patient, and white areas are left in the X-ray film (plate).

3. Invisibility. X-rays cannot be detected by sight, sound or touch. Workers exposed to X-rays must wear a film badge which contains a special film that is exposed by X-rays. The amount of blackness in the film is an indication of the amount of X-rays or gamma rays received by the wearer.

X-rays are used in a variety of ways to detect pathological conditions. The most common use of the diagnostic X-rays is dental, to locate cavities in teeth. Other areas examined are the digestive, nervous, reproductive and endocrine system, the chest and bones.

New Words & Expressions

扫码听
单词

radiology [ˌreɪdɪˈɒlədʒɪ]	n. 放射学,放射线科
cathode [ˈkæθəʊd]	n. 阴极,负极
photographic plate	照相底片,摄影底片
unimpeded [ˌʌnɪmˈpiːdɪd]	adj. 无障碍的,无阻挡的
invisibility [ɪnˌvɪzəˈbɪlətɪ]	n. 看不见,无形
detect [dɪˈtekt]	v. 察觉,发现
film badge	胶片式射线计量器
gamma rays	伽马射线
pathological [ˌpæθəˈlɒdʒɪkəl]	adj. 病理学的,病态的
cavities [ˈkævətɪs]	n. 腔（cavity 的复数形式）

Exercises

Exercise 1. Decide whether the following statements are true (T) or false (F) according to the text.

( ) 1. X-rays are visible waves of energy produced by an energy source.

( ) 2. X-rays have the ability to cause exposure of a photographic plate.

( ) 3. X-rays pass through the different types of substances in the human body.

( ) 4. X-rays can be detected by sight, sound or touch.

( ) 5. The most common use of the diagnostic X-rays is dental, to locate cavities in teeth.

Exercise 2. Fill in the blanks with the words given below, changing the form if necessary.

radiology	impede	penetrate	invisibility
detect	diagnosis	expose	record

1. _____ is the medical specialty concerned with the study of X-rays.

2. _____ testing is typically performed at least twice for this patient.

3. Expert Zhong Nanshan suggests that one such change is an enhancement of the immune system to _____, restrain, and destroy the COVID-19.

Note

4. All the time you are in doubt about your illness, you are fighting against an _____ enemy.

5. A late _____ of disease is likely to cause death.

Exercise 3. Translate the following Chinese sentences into English.

1. 接触 X 射线的工作人员必须佩戴一个胶片式射线计量器,它包含一种被 X 射线照射的特殊胶片。

2. 因此,接触大剂量 X 射线者,在晚年患白血病、甲状腺肿瘤、乳腺癌或其他恶性肿瘤的风险增加。

3. 他发明了一台探测辐射的敏感仪器。

4. X 射线能穿透很多物体。

5. 很难衡量一种化合物到底会如何影响内分泌系统。

Learning More

Ⅰ. Affixes & Roots of Medical Terms

Affixes & Roots	Chinese	More Words
radi(o)-	放射	radiology 放射学;radiation therapy 放射疗法
thyr-	甲状腺	thyroid 甲状腺;thyrocytes 甲状腺细胞
ion(o)-	离子	ionization 离子化;iono music 电离音乐
ultra-	超	ultrastructure 超微结构;ultra violet 紫外线辐射
-therapy	……疗法	radiotherapy 放射疗法;gene therapy 基因疗法

Match the English expressions with the right Chinese phrases.

1. aromatherapy   A. 放射疗法

2. thyroid   B. 离子化

3. radiation therapy   C. 芳香疗法

4. ultrastructure   D. 甲状腺

5. ionization   E. 超微结构

Ⅱ. Vocabulary Expansion

Match the Chinese phrases with the right English expressions.

A. radioscopy	B. radiologist	C. telediagnosis
D. X-ray tomography	E. ultrasonic	F. nonsurgical
G. thyroaplasia	H. physical therapy	I. physician
J. chemotherapy	K. radio dermatitis	L. thermography

1. (　　)放射科医生   (　　)非外科的

2. (　　)超声学   (　　)射线检查法

3. (　　)X 射线体层摄影   (　　)远距离诊断

4. (　　)甲状腺发育不全   (　　)放射性皮炎

5. (　　)化疗   (　　)温度记录法

Note

Practical Writing

Medical History(病史)

病史应该包含以下内容。

1. 患者的基本信息,如姓名、性别、年龄。

2. 现病史。

(1) 病因及诱因。如受凉、饮食、情绪、劳累等。

(2) 主要症状的特点。如发病急缓,出现时间、持续时间、加重或缓解因素,性质,部位等。

(3) 伴随症状(各种疾病的鉴别诊断)。全身状态,即发病以来饮食、睡眠、大小便及体重的变化。

(4) 诊疗经过。发病以来是否到医院检查过,做过哪些治疗,效果如何?

3. 既往史,即药物过敏史、手术史等相关病史。

Sample

Medical History

Feb. 20,2020

Patient:Mr. Mark Thurston

Age:13

Chief complaint:Excessive thirst.

History of present condition:Two or three weeks ago,after meals/eating.

Onset and timing:Go to bathroom six times a day.

Other symptoms:Always tired,looking thin.

Previous occurrence:None.

Past medical history:None.

Medication:None.

Social history:None.

Family history:Mother died of a stroke. Father has a problem of his heart and eyes.

William Smith
Chief Physician
(signature)

Exercise

Write a medical history according to the following information.

【患者:Charmine Plantz,男,24 岁,职业:销售经理,药物史:无,主诉:颈部 1 个月前有无痛性肿块,其他症状:体重减轻、常饿、心跳加速、潮热、腹泻、耳(双耳)嘶嘶声,长期吸烟。】

Extended Knowledge

I. First Aid—Alcohol Poisoning

Step 1 Call Emergency Center immediately to request an ambulance.

Step 2 While you're waiting:

1. Try to keep them sitting up and awake.

2. Give them water if they can drink it.

3. If they have passed out, lie them on their side in the recovery position and check they're breathing properly.

4. Keep them warm.

5. Stay with them.

Warning:

1. Never leave a person alone to "sleep it off". The level of alcohol in a person's blood can continue to rise for up to 30 to 40 minutes after their last drink. This can cause their symptoms to suddenly become much more severe.

2. You also should not try to "sober them up" by giving them coffee or putting them under a cold shower. These methods will not help and may even be dangerous.

II. Knowledge Links

Medical Imaging

The medical device industry is undergoing rapid change as innovation accelerates, new business models emerge, and artificial intelligence (AI) and the Internet of Things create disruptive possibilities in health care. On the innovation front, global annual patent applications related to medical devices have tripled in 10 years, and technology cycle times have halved in just 5 years. Connectivity has exploded. In future, the world will have more than three times as many smart connected devices as people and more and more medical devices and processes contain integrated sensors.

Broadly speaking, medical imaging has benefited from these trends more than other parts of the device industry. That is partly because it generates large digitized data sets that can be subjected to advanced analytics and deep learning. A second reason is that it comprises a full technology stack from hardware to intelligent software, offering ample scope for innovation. Third, improving workflows and the accuracy and speed of diagnostics can deliver measurable benefits in better patient care, reductions in costs and variability, and greater satisfaction for radiologists.

扫码看
答案

Unit 6　Medical Tests

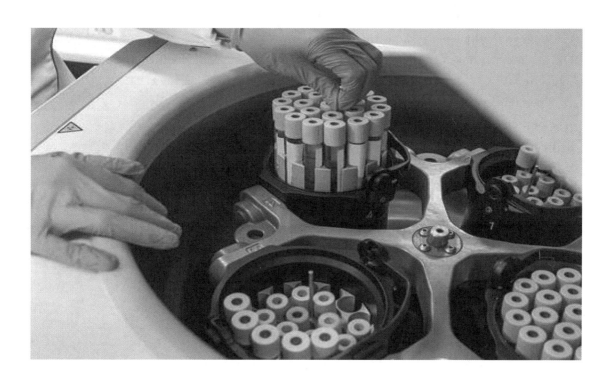

扫码看
PPT

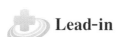 **Lead-in**

Medical tests, as diagnosing tools, play an important role in getting early warning of unforeseen diseases or disorders. After all, there is no better way to assure yourself of being absolutely healthy and perfectly fit. It is necessary for individuals to learn some knowledge about medical tests.

Thinking & Talking

1. Please list names of some medical tests that you know.
2. Why are medical tests necessary for people?

Focus Listening

扫码听
对话 1

Conversation 1

Directions: *You will hear a conversation between a patient, Wang Hua and a nurse, Miss Chen.*

 Note

Wang Hua was admitted late yesterday afternoon with a lump in her right breast. She's going to have a fine-needle biopsy this afternoon. Now she is talking to Miss Chen, her nurse in charge on the ward. Listen carefully and fill in the blanks according to the conversation.

A: Excuse me, Miss Chen, can I have a word with you?

B: Sure.

A: I'm having a test this afternoon and I don't know what 1. _____ it is. I'm worried about it. Could you explain it to me?

B: I'm sure you are clear about your problem.

A: I've got a lump in my right 2. _____ .

B: OK. Well, you are having a fine-needle biopsy.

A: Could you tell me more about the test?

B: They use a syringe and they 3. _____ on it and get some of the fluid and some of the cells. After that they 4. _____ to a pathology and cytology lab to check on the cells.

A: When can I get the results?

B: You probably won't find out until tomorrow or later than that.

A: I am wondering whether I need an 5. _____ if the results turn out to be 6. _____ ?

B: Well, if the results come back as all clear, then you won't need an operation.

A: OK and if it's not all clear?

B: Well, your doctor has 7. _____ you ultrasound test which is to be done tomorrow. So we shall wait for the results of both those tests. The doctor will decide whether you need an operation or not according to the results.

A: So basically we shall 8. _____ .

B: Yeah, unfortunately, it is, yes.

A: I got it. Thanks for your explanation.

New Words & Expressions

lump [lʌmp]	n.	块,肿块
syringe [sɪˈrɪndʒ]	n.	注射器
fluid [ˈfluːɪd]	n.	液体,流体,液
cell [sel]	n.	细胞
pathology [pəˈθɒlədʒɪ]	n.	病理学
cytology [saɪˈtɒlədʒɪ]	n.	细胞学
ultrasound [ˈʌltrəsaʊnd]	n.	超声波扫描检查

Conversation 2

Directions: *You will hear a conversation between a patient, Ms. Wang and a nurse, Miss Li. Ms. Wang is a 43-year-old woman who is now in her 31st week of pregnancy. She has been hospitalized recently for occasional headache. She was diagnosed as hypertensive disorders in pregnancy. Now she complains that her headache is much more serious when the nurse Miss Li comes into the ward. Listen to the conversation carefully and then choose the best answer for each of the following questions.*

1. Is Ms. Wang suffering from headache now? _____ .

   A. Yes, she is   B. No, she isn't   C. It's not mentioned

2. Which of the test has not been mentioned in the dialogue? _____ .

A. Blood test   B. Urine test   C. Stool test

3. What are the symptoms of hypertensive disorders in pregnancy? _____ .

A. High blood pressure   B. Edema   C. Both A and B

4. Can the nurse give Ms. Wang medicine now? _____ .

A. Yes, she can   B. No, she can't   C. It's not mentioned

5. How about the patient's blood pressure? _____ .

A. Higher than the normal

B. Lower than the normal

C. Normal

New Words & Expressions

pregnancy ['pregnənsɪ]	n. 妊娠,怀孕,孕期
hospitalize ['hɒspɪtəlaɪz]	v. 住院治疗
diagnose ['daɪəgnəʊz]	v. 诊断(疾病)
hypertensive disorders in pregnancy	妊娠高血压
edema [ɪ'diːmə]	n. 水肿
bend [bend]	v. (使四肢等)弯曲
urine test	尿检
blood test	血液检查
protein ['prəʊtiːn]	n. 蛋白质
anemic [ə'nɪmɪk]	adj. 贫血的,患贫血症的

扫码听
单词

Group Discussion & Role Playing

1. Discuss with your partner. Change the patient types or demands and redesign the conversation.

2. Display the conversation you've made.

3. After one group finishes the performance, others make comments.

Intensive Reading

Medical Tests

A medical test refers to a kind of medical procedure performed to detect, diagnose, or monitor diseases, disease processes, susceptibility, and to determine a course of treatment. It is related to clinical chemistry and molecular diagnostics, and the procedures are typically performed in a medical laboratory. Medical tests are used for a variety of purposes. When receiving patients, a doctor may order these tests as a routine checkup, to check for certain diseases or to monitor their health. They work as an employment requisite in some instances.

扫码听
课文

Note

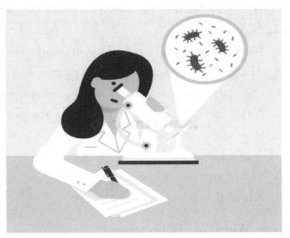

Generally speaking, common medical tests that we are familiar with include blood test, pathology test, blood sugar test, genetic test, cholesterol test and endoscopy test. Medical tests can be classified into different types based on different standards. According to the sample being tested, medical tests are divided into blood test, urine test, stool test and sputum test. Such common tests mentioned above include: measuring the blood sugar in a person suspected of having diabetes, after periods of increased urination; taking a complete blood count of an individual experiencing a high fever, to check for a bacterial infection; monitoring electrocardiogram readings on a patient suffering chest pain, to diagnose any heart irregularities.

While it is true that some medical testing procedures pose certain health risks and even require the subject to be anesthetized, most common medical tests like blood test or pregnancy test pose little or no direct risk.

New Words & Expressions

monitor [ˈmɒnɪtə(r)]	v. 监视,检查,跟踪调查
susceptibility [səˌseptəˈbɪlətɪ]	n. 易受影响的特性,易感性
clinical [ˈklɪnɪkl]	adj. 临床的
molecular [məˈlekjʊlə(r)]	adj. 分子的
requisite [ˈrekwɪzɪt]	n. 必需的
instance [ˈɪnstəns]	n. 例子,实例
blood sugar test	血糖测试
genetic [dʒəˈnetɪk] test	基因测试
cholesterol [kəˈlestərɒl] test	胆固醇测试
endoscopy [enˈdɒskəpɪ] test	内镜检查
sample [ˈsɑːmpl]	n. (化验的)取样,样本
sputum [ˈspjuːtəm]	n. (尤指因疾病咳出的)痰
urination [jʊərɪˈneɪʃən]	n. 排尿
complete blood count	全血计数,血常规
irregularity [ɪˌregjʊˈlærətɪ]	n. 不规则或者是无规律的事物
pose [pəʊz]	v. 造成,引起,产生
pregnancy test	孕检

Note

Exercises

Exercise 1. Decide whether the following statements are true (T) or false (F) according to the text.

(　　) 1. Medical tests can be classified based on only one standard.

(　　) 2. Measuring the blood sugar is necessary for a person suspected of having diabetes.

(　　) 3. All medical testing procedures pose certain health risks for people.

(　　) 4. Blood test only apply to people who are having a fever.

(　　) 5. Medical tests can be the only requisite for an employment.

Exercise 2. Fill in the blanks with the words given below, changing the form if necessary.

blood sugar	pregnancy	genetic	sputum
anesthetics	diagnosis	infection	pose

1. If it's 5 or higher, you're at high risk for diabetes. See your doctor for a _____ test.

2. If you really can't wait, a home _____ test may give you results by the end of the week, but if it's negative and you still don't get your period, try again in a few days.

3. They learn how to _____ and manage common illnesses like colds, or chronic problems such as diabetes and heart disease.

4. The findings also raise the possibility of developing a _____ test to predict an individual's chances of living past 100.

5. Operations without _____ usually had to be done and the person operated on could feel all the pain.

Exercise 3. Translate the following Chinese sentences into English.

1. 医学检验根据样本分为血液检测、尿液检测、粪便检测和痰液检测。

2. 常见的医学检验包括血液检查、病理检查、血糖检查、基因检测、胆固醇检测和内镜检查。

3. 医学检验通常在医学实验室进行。

4. 医学检验有助于医生检测、诊断和监测疾病。

5. 高热患者被要求做一个全血计数来确认是否有细菌感染。

Learning More

Ⅰ. Affixes & Roots of Medical Terms

Affixes & Roots	Chinese	More Words
electro-	电的	electromagnetic 电磁的
hyper-	高于,超过	hypertension 高血压;hypertensive 高血压的
hypo-	过低的	hypotension 低血压;hypotensive 低血压的
cardio-	心	cardiovascular 心血管的;cardiopulmonary 心肺的
-gist	专家	cardiologist 心脏病医生;radiologist 放射科医生
-tomy	切除术	appendectomy 阑尾切除术;tonsillectomy 扁桃体切除术
endo-	内	endoscopy 内镜检查;endovascular 血管内的
-logy	学科	pathology 病理学;cardiology 心脏病学

Note

Match the English expressions with the right Chinese phrases.

1. hypotension   A. 心脏病医生
2. cytology   B. 专家
3. appendectomy   C. 低血压
4. cardiopulmonary   D. 阑尾切除术
5. cardiologist   E. 心肺的
6. specialist   F. 细胞学

Ⅱ. Vocabulary Expansion

Match the Chinese phrases with the right English expressions.

A. sample	B. blood sugar test	C. symptom
D. infection	E. dose	F. biopsy
G. pregnancy test	H. clinical	I. diagnosis
J. diabetes	K. urination	L. anesthetics

1. (   )糖尿病   (   )诊断
2. (   )样本   (   )血糖检查
3. (   )妊娠检查   (   )麻醉剂
4. (   )剂量   (   )排尿
5. (   )感染   (   )症状

Practical Writing

Disease Description(疾病描述)

描述疾病时应该包含以下内容:疾病名称、疾病定义、疾病初期症状及主要症状、疾病并发症、疾病原因、疾病诊断手段和治疗方案。

描述疾病的基本情况需要详细、精准,不得加入个人观点。以题目提到的内容为基础,不要随意添加。题目所提供的信息多以词组呈现,为写出连贯的句子和文章,学生可添加适当动词,如 determine、suspect、prescribe、uncover、occur 等,也可以通过改变单词的词性使表达更为贴切,如将 shortness 改为 short,将 abnormal 改为 abnormally 等。另外,可以巧妙地使用关联词来增强段落的连贯性,以下的范文中主要使用了一些常见的关联词,如 however、but、unless、once 等。

Sample

Acute Appendicitis

Definition:acute inflammation of the appendix

First symptoms:pain all over the abdomen, or only in the upper abdomen, or about the navel, fever (T < 38 ℃)

The most prominent symptom:pain in the right lower quadrant

Complications:appendix abscess, ruptured appendix, peritonitis (T > 38 ℃)

Cause:appendix becomes blocked, often by stool, a foreign body, or cancer

Diagnosis: symptoms, a physical exam, blood test and urine test

Treatment: surgery to remove the appendix

Acute appendicitis is the acute inflammation of the appendix. The first symptom of the disease is pain all over the abdomen, or only in the upper abdomen, or about the navel. However, pain in the right lower quadrant is the most prominent symptom of the disease. Fever is present, but usually does not exceed 38 ℃ unless there are complications such as appendix abscess, ruptured appendix and peritonitis.

Appendicitis occurs when the appendix becomes blocked, often by stool, a foreign body, or cancer. The doctor bases an appendicitis diagnosis on symptoms, a physical exam, blood test and urine test to check for signs of infection. Once a diagnosis of the disease is made, western medicine will usually prescribe surgery to remove the appendix.

Exercise

Please write a disease description according to the information given below.

Shock
Definition: sudden or acute failure of the circulation
Symptoms in early stage: losing consciousness, abnormal temperature
Symptoms in advanced stage: deep coma, gastrointestinal problems arise
Complications: respiratory distress or failure, intestinal ischemia, stroke, etc.
Cause: inadequate substrate for aerobic cellular respiration
Diagnosis: upon tests (X-rays, blood test)
Prompt treatment: fluid resuscitation with an I. V.

Extended Knowledge

Ⅰ. First Aid—Spinal Injury

Step 1 Get help.

Call 911 or emergency medical help.

Step 2 Keep the person still.

Place heavy towels or rolled sheets on both sides of the neck or hold the head and neck to prevent movement.

Step 3 Avoid moving the head or neck.

Provide as much first aid as possible without moving the person's head or neck. If the person shows no signs of circulation (breathing, coughing or movement), begin CPR, but do not tilt the head back to open the airway. Use your fingers to gently grasp the jaw and lift it forward. If the person has no pulse, begin chest compression.

Step 4 Keep helmet on.

If the person is wearing a helmet, don't remove it.

Step 5 Don't roll alone.

If you must roll the person because he or she is vomiting, choking on blood or because you have to make sure the person is still breathing, you need at least one other person. With one of you at the head and another along the side of the injured person, work together to keep the person's head, neck and back aligned while rolling the person onto one side.

II. Knowledge Links

Egg Allergy

Egg allergies are most common in young children. As the children grow up, they may stop experiencing allergic reactions to egg proteins. The symptoms of egg allergies usually occur a few minutes after you have consumed eggs. Most people experience mild allergic symptoms. The problem with an egg allergy is that any food product containing eggs can trigger it off.

An allergist or an allergy specialist will be able to administer certain tests to check for possible allergies. You have to undergo several medical tests before the allergy is actually identified. The allergist will first perform a physical examination before performing any egg allergy tests. The doctor will also ask you several questions about your allergy symptoms to get a more accurate background of your condition. After these initial tests are done, a skin test may be performed. The doctor will get you to do a prick test. This test involves exposing your pricked skin to several different foods. After the skin is exposed to these foods and the proteins in them, the doctor looks for any allergic reactions such as inflammation, rashes, and formation of hives on the skin. The doctor may also look for other allergic reactions such as respiratory or digestive discomfort. To prepare for this test, you have to stop taking certain medications. Cold medications as well as antidepressants may also have to be discontinued for a few days before your test. Blood test may also be performed to look for any specific antibodies that may indicate an allergic reaction in the body.

扫码看
答案

Unit 7　Internal Medicine

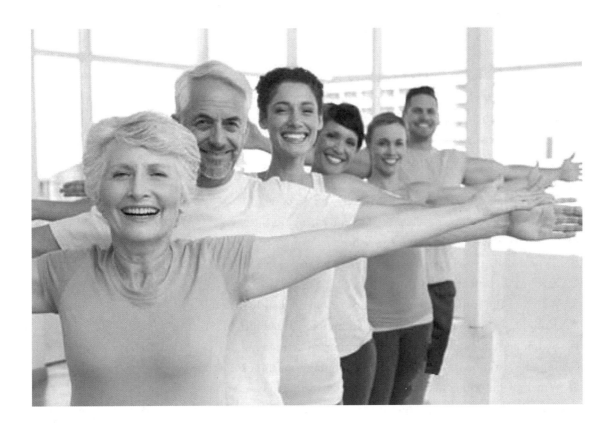

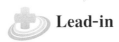 Lead-in

Internal medicine is the medical specialty dealing with the prevention, diagnosis, and treatment of adult diseases. It is the branch of medicine that deals with the diagnosis and nonsurgical treatment of diseases of the internal organs, especially in adults. Physicians specializing in internal medicine are called internists, who are skilled in the management of patients who have undifferentiated or multi-system disease processes. Internists care for hospitalized and ambulatory patients and may play a major role in teaching and research.

Thinking & Talking

1. What are the safety hazards in medical care?
2. Can you share any nursing strategies for elderly inpatients in internal medicine?

Note

49

Focus Listening

Conversation 1

扫码听
对话 1

Directions: *You will hear a conversation between a doctor and a patient with a weight problem. Choose the best answer for each of the following questions.*

1. The patient should take care of his weight problem because _____.
A. his BMI is 33.8　　　　B. his BMI is 38.2　　　　C. his BMI is 32.8

2. What is BMI? _____.
A. A person's weight in grams divided by height in centimeters squared
B. A person's weight in kilograms divided by height in meters squared
C. A person's height in meters squared divided by weight in kilograms

3. An adult is considered obese because _____.
A. he is 50 and older, having a BMI: 25-29.9
B. he is 30 and older, having a BMI: greater than 35
C. he is 35 and older, having a BMI: greater than 30

4. Which of the following diseases are caused by obesity? _____.
A. Insulin resistance, hypertension, headache
B. Type 2 diabetes, hypertension, sleep apnea
C. Stroke, Type 1 diabetes, heart attack

5. Which of the following exercises are recommended by the doctor? _____.
A. Running, stationary bicycling, walking on a treadmill
B. Swimming, mountain climbing, jogging on a treadmill
C. Jogging, stationary bicycling, stair climbing machines

6. Which of the following is true according to the conversation? _____.
A. In order to lose weight, the patient has done exercise for weeks but it didn't work
B. The patient's parents experienced the same problem as the patient himself
C. Despite weight problem, the patient's blood pressure remains steady recently

New Words & Expressions

扫码听
单词

BMI (Body Mass Index)	n. 体重指数
obese [əʊˈbiːs]	adj. 肥胖的,过胖的
genetic [dʒəˈnetɪk]	adj. 遗传的,基因的
insulin resistance	胰岛素耐受性
sleep apnea	睡眠呼吸暂停
metabolism [məˈtæbəlɪzəm]	n. 新陈代谢

Conversation 2

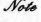

Note

Directions: *You will hear a conversation between Mrs. King and a doctor. Mrs. King starts to lose her memory. She comes to Dr. Williams for help. Listen carefully and decide whether the following statements are true (T) or false (F).*

( ) 1. It is the first time that Dr. Williams has met Mrs. King in recent years.

( ) 2. Dr. Williams has taken over Dr. Wang's practice for several years.

( ) 3. Mrs. King's house is located on the High Street.

( ) 4. According to her memory, Mrs. King stayed with her father after she got married.

( ) 5. Mrs. King can exactly remember her age.

New Words & Expressions

retire [rɪˈtaɪə(r)]	v. 退休,离开
recall [rɪˈkɔːl]	v. 召回,回想起
take over	接管,接收
no doubt	无疑地,很可能地

Group Discussion & Role Playing

1. Discuss with your partner. Change the patient types or demands and redesign the conversation.

2. Display the conversation you've made.

3. After one group finishes the performance, others make comments.

Intensive Reading

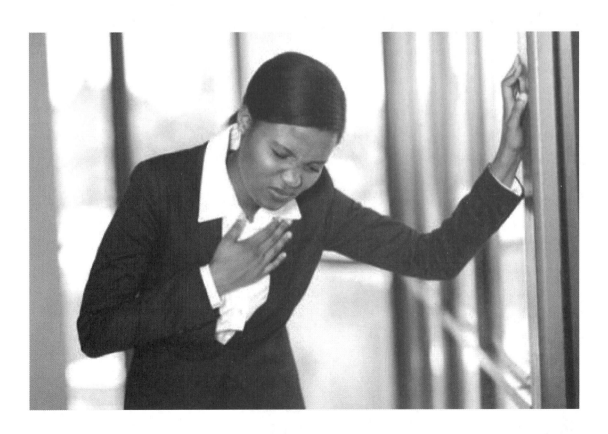

Broken Heart Syndrome

Broken heart syndrome, also called stress-induced cardiomyopathy, can strike even if you're healthy.

Women are more likely than men to experience the sudden, intense chest pain—the reaction to a surge of stress hormones—that can be caused by an emotionally stressful event. It could be the death of a loved one or even a divorce, breakup, etc. It could even happen after a good shock.

Broken heart syndrome may be misdiagnosed as a heart attack because the symptoms and test results are similar. In fact, tests show dramatic changes in heart rate and substances in the blood, which are typical symptoms of a heart attack. But unlike a heart attack, there's no evidence of blocked heart arteries in broken heart syndrome.

In broken heart syndrome, a part of your heart temporarily enlarges and doesn't pump well, while the rest of your heart functions normally or with even more forceful contractions. Researchers are just starting to learn the causes, and how to diagnose and treat it.

The bad news: Broken heart syndrome can lead to severe, short-term heart muscle failure.

The good news: Broken heart syndrome is usually curable. Most people who experience it make a full recovery within a few weeks, and they're at low risk for it happening again (although in rare cases it can be fatal).

What to look out: signs and symptoms.

The most common signs and symptoms of broken heart syndrome are angina (chest pain) and shortness of breath. You can experience these things even if you have no history of heart disease.

Arrhythmias (irregular heartbeats) or cardiogenic shock also may occur with broken heart syndrome. Cardiogenic shock is a condition in which a suddenly weakened heart can't pump enough blood to meet the body's needs, and it can be fatal if it isn't treated right away. When people die from heart attacks, cardiogenic shock is the most common cause of death.

New Words & Expressions

syndrome [ˈsɪndrəʊm]	n. 综合症状,并发症状
cardiomyopathy [ˌkɑːdɪəʊmaɪˈɒpəθɪ]	n. (尤指原发性的)心肌症,心肌病
surge [sɜːdʒ]	n. 猛增,急剧上升
misdiagnose [mɪsˈdaɪəgnəʊz]	v. 错误判断,误诊
artery [ˈɑːtərɪ]	n. 动脉,干道,主流
forceful [ˈfɔːsfʊl]	adj. 强有力的,有说服力的,坚强的
fatal [ˈfeɪtəl]	adj. 致命的,重大的,毁灭性的
curable [ˈkjʊərəbl]	adj. 可治愈的,可医治的,可矫正的
angina [ænˈdʒaɪnə]	n. 心绞痛
arrhythmia [əˈrɪðmɪə]	n. 心律失常
cardiogenic [ˌkɑːdɪəʊˈdʒenɪk]	adj. 心源性的,心脏发生的
broken heart syndrome	心碎综合征
stress-induced cardiomyopathy	应激性心肌病
stress hormone	应激激素
heart attack	心脏病发作
in rhythm	有节奏地

lead to	导致,通向
at risk	处于危险中
meet one's needs	符合某人的需要

Exercises

Exercise 1. Decide whether the following statements are true (T) or false (F) according to the text.

(　　) 1. When a woman found her husband dating with a beautiful young lady in a romantic restaurant，she might experience the sudden，intense chest pain.

(　　) 2. The symptoms and test results of broken heart syndrome are quite different from a real heart attack.

(　　) 3. Heart arteries can be found blocked in the patients with broken heart syndrome.

(　　) 4. When broken heart syndrome strikes，the whole heart will temporarily enlarge but pump well.

(　　) 5. The patients with broken heart syndrome can be fully recovered through the reasonable treatment，while they're at high risk for it happening again.

Exercise 2. Fill in the blanks with the words given below, changing the form if necessary.

| lead to | forceful | surge | meet one's needs |
| curable | stress | fatal | risk |

1. Aging itself might be seen as something _____, the way you would treat high blood pressure or a vitamin deficiency.

2. I think her headache is caused by _____.

3. Wearing a helmet increases the chance of people taking more _____.

4. The nearest community sports in spare time has become one of the main ways to _____ in sports.

5. Americans view five hours of TV each day，and while we know that spending so much time sitting passively can _____ obesity and other diseases.

Exercise 3. Translate the following Chinese sentences into English.

1. 营养不良能反映贫穷、战争、饥荒以及疾病等问题。
2. 这些事实充分说明,这种疾病总体上是可控和可治的。
3. 患者有高血压、糖尿病、冠心病等基础疾病。
4. 这是所有病毒中最致命、最具毁灭性的。
5. 对于任何治疗,术后恢复不仅取决于手术过程,还取决于术后护理。

Learning More

Ⅰ. Affixes & Roots of Medical Terms

Affixes & Roots	Chinese	More Words
cardio-	心	cardiology 心脏病学;cardiopulmonary 与心肺有关的
mis-	错误的,不好的	misdiagnose 误诊;misdirect 误导
sym-	连,共同	symptom 症状;sympathy 同情,慰问
syn-	类似,共同	syndrome 综合征;syndication 企业联合组织

Note

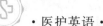

Match the English expressions with the right Chinese phrases.

1. cardiomyopathy   A. 心碎综合征

2. hormone   B. 心源性休克

3. broken heart syndrome   C. 心绞痛

4. cardiogenic shock   D. 心肌病

5. angina   E. 心律失常

6. arrhythmias   F. 激素，荷尔蒙

Ⅱ. Vocabulary Expansion

Match the Chinese phrases with the right English expressions.

A. heart muscle	B. contraction	C. win the lottery
D. heart attack	E. artery	F. heart function
G. cause of death	H. stroke	I. shortness of breath
J. chest pain	K. nitroglycerin	L. heart beat

1. (   )心脏功能   (   )心跳

2. (   )心脏病发作   (   )呼吸急促

3. (   )硝酸甘油   (   )动脉

4. (   )死因   (   )脑卒中

5. (   )心肌   (   )收缩

6. (   )中彩票   (   )胸痛

Practical Writing

Nursing Plan(护理计划)

护理计划是针对护理诊断制定的具体护理措施，是指导护理行为的纲领性文件。它必须围绕患者的病情，通过能够实施的护理方法，具体指导临床护理实践。

护理计划的主要内容包含三个部分，第一部分描述患者目前的基本情况，第二部分描述与此病患沟通交流的方法，第三部分为沟通的结果。

Read the following background information. Write a nursing plan for the patient.

Patient name	Samuel Johnson
Age	70
Marital status	widower
Next of kin	two children who both live in other countries
On admission	insomnia（2 years）, bad headaches, breathlessness, lack of appetite, hypertension, moderate generalized weakness, uninterested in anything
Impression	depression

护理计划属于说明文，请根据上述表格中所提供的信息写一份护理计划。在写作此文时应注意：

第一部分的基本情况描写应基于表格的信息，写作时需使用正确的标点符号、适当的连词将表中的词或词组连成句子，必要时进行顺序调整，使句子语意连贯、重点突出。

第二部分为护理此病患的解决方法。针对第一部分中总结的典型问题（年龄大、无亲人在身边、抑郁、长期失眠等），提出 2 至 3 种护理方法，并举例子说明。

第三部分为结果，总结上述护理带来的良好结果。

根据内容判断，写作时应运用一般现在时，还应做到语法结构正确，上下文过渡自然，使用多种句型结构和丰富的词组。

Sample

Nursing Plan

Mr. Johnson, a 70-year-old widower, has been diagnosed with depression. Both of his two children live in other countries, so he leads a lonely life. He has been suffering from insomnia for two years, and gradually developed bad headaches, breathlessness, lack of appetite, hypertension and moderate generalized weakness, which make him lose interest in anything around him.

When treating patients with depression like Mr. Johnson, firstly, I think we should make clear of their preferences, especially some eccentric living habits, and choose proper ways to satisfy their different requirements. Secondly, we should be patient and respectfully enough in getting along with them, because depressed elderly patients tend to be oversensitive, stubborn and irritable. For example, when they lose control of their emotions, we had better calm them down with expertise and words of comfort.

To sum up, only when professional care is provided can the patients achieve a sense of trust, which would facilitate their communication with us, and consequently improve the therapeutic efficacy.

Exercise

Please write a nursing plan according to the information given below.

【Marie Thomas，女性，35 岁，体重 92 公斤，有心脏病史，喝酒，抽烟，从不锻炼。请仿照例文给这位病患写一份合理的护理计划，建议戒酒戒烟，适当运动，合理饮食。】

Patient name	Marie Thomas
Age	35
Weight	92 kg
Next of kin	Her mother has angina and her father died of heart attack.
Medical history	a history of heart disease, drinking, smoking, and never exercising
On admission	no appetite, breathing problem (1 year), shooting pains in her left arm (3 weeks)
Nursing advice	stop drinking and smoking, do regular exercise, eat a low cholesterol diet

Extended Knowledge

Ⅰ. First Aid—Sunstroke or heatstroke

Step 1 Call for help.

Call to get an ambulance as quickly as possible. Ask everyone to bring you as much water as possible, if there isn't much nearby.

Note

Step 2 Get the person to a cooler area.

If there's a building nearby, aim for that. Anywhere with plenty of air conditioners and water is perfect. If a building isn't available, bring the person to a well-shaded area.

Step 3 Get the water flowing.

If the person is still conscious, get him or her to drink water. If there's a bathtub available, fill it with cool water and put it on the person's body. Focus on the face, neck and chest.

Step 4 Fan the person.

Getting moving air over the person cools him or her down. Use anything, a towel or sheet, a shirt, your hands, or a piece of board.

Ⅱ. Knowledge Links

Psychiatric Nursing

Psychiatric nurses confront both opportunities and risks at present and in the future as well. The future challenges psychiatric nursing to find creative responses to decreasing public support, the importance of nursing care in treatment of the mentally ill and the socially deviant will be confirmed through continued commitment to progress in research, practice and education.

Mental health-psychiatric nursing needs to confront two challenges in the coming decades. First, nurses must actively participate in establishing the conditions under which interpersonal treatment methods are effective in preventing or relieving mental disorders. Second, nurses must actively participate in establishing the conditions under which mental health-psychiatric nursing practice interacts with the treatment methods.

What is the best way to care for an individual who is mentally ill? Through the ages this care had been the product of two different traditions, one stressing a need to appease in some way magic or supernatural forces and the other attempting to understand through rational methods the causes and cure of the disease.

扫码看
答案

Note

Unit 8　Surgery

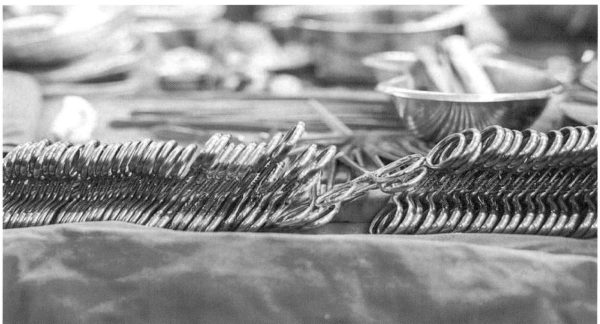

扫码看
PPT

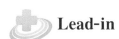 **Lead-in**

Surgery is an important part of the clinical medicine. It mainly researches the etiology, occurrence, development, diagnosis and treatment of surgical disease. Surgery often deals with trauma, various thoracic and abdominal emergencies, malformations, tumors, organ transportation, etc. In clinical application, it has a close relationship with anesthesiology, special nursing, radiation, oncology and other medical specialties.

In the surgical department, nurses take various responsibilities. They assist surgeons during both routine and difficult surgical procedures and they look after patients before, during and after these procedures. The job requires that the nurses possess strong analytical, technical, administrative and organizational skills in addition to communication skills normally associated with the nursing profession.

Thinking & Talking

1. What does surgery often deal with?
2. Whom might a surgical nurse work with?

Note

Focus Listening

Conversation 1

扫码听
对话 1

Directions：*You will hear a conversation between <u>Andrew</u> and <u>a doctor</u>. Andrew is brought to the hospital for a sports accident. Listen to the conversation carefully and decide whether the following statements are true（T）or false（F）.*

（　　）1. Andrew is going to lose his injured foot.

（　　）2. The injured foot could move a little.

（　　）3. The doctor rates the pain as 8.

（　　）4. The doctor orders a wrap and a wheelchair for Andrew.

New Words & Expressions

扫码听
单词

pulse ［pʌls］	n. 脉搏
fracture ［ˈfræktʃə(r)］	n. 骨折
wrap ［ræp］	n. 包扎
crutch ［krʌtʃ］	n. 拐杖，支柱
ambulation ［æmbjʊˈleɪʃən］	n. 移动，步行

Conversation 2

Directions：*You will hear a conversation between <u>Andrew</u> and <u>a nurse</u>. Listen carefully and choose the right answer for each of the following questions.*

扫码听
对话 2

1. How does Andrew feel after the wrap? ＿＿＿＿＿.

A. He feels dizzy　　　　B. He feels better　　　　C. He can feel his pulse

2. Is Andrew able to stand up by himself? ＿＿＿＿＿.

A. Yes，he is　　　　B. No，he isn't　　　　C. It depends

3. When using the crutches，where should Andrew put his weight? ＿＿＿＿＿.

A. On his feet　　　　B. On his arms　　　　C. On the handles

4. When standing with crutches，where should Andrew put his weight? ＿＿＿＿＿.

A. On the good leg　　　　B. On the injured foot　　　　C. On the handles

New Words & Expressions

扫码听
单词

dizzy ［ˈdɪzɪ］	adj. 头晕的，眩晕的
adjust ［əˈdʒʌst］	v. 调整，使适合
handle ［ˈhændl］	n. 柄，把手

Note

Group Discussion & Role Playing

1. Discuss with your partner. Change the patient types or demands and redesign the conversation.

2. Display the conversation you've made.

3. After one group finishes the performance, others make comments.

Intensive Reading

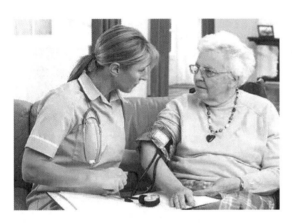 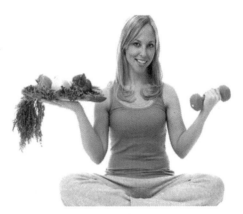

扫码听
课文

How to Handle Worry During Watchful Waiting

If you've been diagnosed with cancer, it's likely that your oncologist will recommend a period of "watchful waiting". Watchful waiting can be psychologically challenging, which depends on your diagnosis and time in active treatment (chemo, radiation or surgery).

You may worry that cancer will grow and spread while you are waiting; you may feel anxiety that the doctors are "doing nothing" to fight cancer while you're waiting; or you may feel stuck, unable to get back into your regular life until you know the results of the scans or tests that will happen at the end of watchful waiting. Hearing about other people's experiences can help you form a coping strategy that works for you. Beth's story may give you some useful insights.

Beth was diagnosed with a stage I breast cancer in her left breast, which was treated with surgery and radiation. During a routine postoperative examination, a mammogram revealed a potentially concerning spot on the right breast. To her surprise, instead of suggesting immediate active treatment of the right breast, her oncologist recommended watchful waiting for 3 months and a repeat mammogram. Beth voiced her concern to her oncologist, "In three months that spot could be cancer and start spreading all over the breast!" Beth's oncologist explained that since the spot had been stable on previous mammograms, it was very unlikely to be an active cancer site and reassured her that there were several things she could do to fight cancer over the next three months.

The cancer fighting plan during watchful waiting for Beth included an anti-inflammatory diet and a safe movement program. She replaced red meat and sodas with beans, vegetables and bubbly water and joined a dance group for exercise three days a week. Losing weight and doing exercises not only

Note

improved Beth's body image, but also diminished her worry about cancer growing or spreading, "I am doing everything I can to stay healthy, and that feels good!"

The watchful waiting period often comes with some worry, but with attention to thinking patterns and self-care, watchful waiting could be a time that you really focus on meaningful activities instead of being a cancer patient.

New Words & Expressions

扫码听
单词

oncologist [ɒŋˈkɒlədʒɪst]	n. 肿瘤学家,肿瘤师
psychologically [ˌsaɪkəˈlɒdʒɪklɪ]	adv. 心理上地,心理学地
challenging [ˈtʃælɪndʒɪŋ]	adj. 挑战性的
chemo [ˈkiːməʊ]	n. 化疗,化学疗法
radiation [ˌreɪdɪˈeɪʃən]	n. 辐射,放射物
surgery [ˈsɜːdʒərɪ]	n. 外科学,外科手术
strategy [ˈstrætədʒɪ]	n. 战略,策略
mammogram [ˈmæməgræm]	n. 乳房 X 线照片
reveal [rɪˈviːl]	v. 显示,透露
reassure [ˌriːəˈʃʊə(r)]	v. 使安心,再次确保
anti-inflammatory [ˌæntɪɪnˈflæmətərɪ]	adj. 抗炎的
diminish [dɪˈmɪnɪʃ]	v. 使减少,使变小
watchful waiting	观察等待

Exercises

Exercise 1. Decide whether the following statements are true (T) or false (F) according to the text.

(　　) 1. During the watchful waiting period, there is nothing the patient can do to fight cancer.

(　　) 2. Watchful waiting is not a psychologically challenging period for Beth.

(　　) 3. Beth's doctor told her that the concerning spot was not an active cancer site.

(　　) 4. Beth lived a healthy life over the watchful waiting time.

(　　) 5. The patient is suggested to focus on meaningful life activities over the watchful waiting time.

Exercise 2. Fill in the blanks with the words given below, changing the form if necessary.

diagnose　　　　oncologist　　　　watchful waiting　　　　psychologically
reveal　　　　reassure　　　　anti-inflammatory　　　　diminish

1. The old man was _____ as having flu.

2. While holding off on medical or surgical treatment, _____ is a reasonable plan for them.

3. Some people find it _____ difficult to accept the fact that they have cancer.

4. A survey of the American diet has _____ that a growing number of people are overweight.

5. As an _____, he is determined to treat patients as he would wish to be treated.

Exercise 3. Translate the following Chinese sentences into English.

1. 王先生在车祸中失去了一条腿,他从心理上很难接受这一事实。

2. 医生帮她制订了一个消炎饮食计划对抗癌症。

3. 确诊癌症后,她接受了放疗和化疗。

4. 请尽快找出导致这次测试准确性降低的原因。

5. 在观察等待期,患者需要做一些必要的身体检查。

Note

60

Learning More

I. Affixes & Roots of Medical Terms

Affixes & Roots	Chinese	More Words
radi(o)-	放射	radiation 辐射；radioactivity 放射性
psych(o)-	精神，心理	psychology 心理学；psychiatry 精神病学
mammo(o)-	乳房	mammogram 乳房 X 线照片；mammogen 乳腺发育激素
-gram	图，描记图	hemogram 血象；electrocardiogram 心电图
anti-	抗，防止	anti-inflammatory 抗炎的；antibiotics 抗生素

Match the English expressions with the right Chinese phrases.

1. electrocardiogram   A. 抗炎的
2. psychology   B. 乳房 X 线照片
3. radiology   C. 心电图
4. mammogram   D. 心理学
5. anti-inflammatory   E. 放射学

II. Vocabulary Expansion

Match the Chinese phrases with the right English expressions.

A. diagnose	B. fracture	C. pulse
D. crutch	E. watchful waiting	F. wrap
G. active treatment	H. spread	I. ambulation
J. reveal	K. radiation treatment	L. surgery

1. ( )外科手术   ( )诊断
2. ( )拐杖   ( )观察等待
3. ( )放疗   ( )扩散
4. ( )脉搏   ( )骨折
5. ( )步行   ( )积极治疗

Practical Writing

Handover Report(交班报告)

护士交班报告书写要求如下。

1. 填写眉栏及文件上所列项目：年、月、日，原有病员数，入院、出院、转出病员数，危重、手术、分娩、死亡病员数。

2. 根据下列顺序，按床号先后书写报告：出院、转出、死亡、新入、转入、手术、病危、病重、备手术。内容简明扼要，表述准确无误，突出重点。

3. 格式：床号、姓名书写在同一行，下一行写主要诊断、手术、转入等特殊标识。

4. 交班内容：①出院患者报告床号、姓名、诊断、出院时间和转归情况；②转出患者报告床号、姓名、诊断、转出时间和转入科室；③死亡患者报告简要的病情变化、抢救经过和死亡时间；④新入院（转入）患者报告病人床号、姓名、性别、年龄、入院或转入的疾病诊断、入院时间、生命体征、病情和主要治疗护理措施等；⑤当日手术患者报告手术名称、麻醉方式、回病房时间、生命体征、伤口及各种引流管情况、疼痛、采取的主要治疗和护理措施等；⑥预备手术患者报告拟手术时间、名称、麻醉方式、术前准备情况等；⑦病危及病重患者简要报告病情、生命体征及治疗、护理情况。

Sample

Handover Report

Date：Mar. 14，2020

Bed No. Name Diagnosis / Pathogenic condition general report	Total number of patients：25
	Admitted：1　　Discharged：1　　Transferred out：0 Transferred in：0　　Operated：1　　Labor：0 New born：0　　Apogee：0　　Death：0
Bed 2 Liu Li	Discharged at 9：00 a. m.
Bed 9 Wang Qiang	Admitted at 11：30 a. m.
Bed 18 Yuan Nan CA of colon	Male，50 years old，under Dr. Xu. Had a hemicolectomy and now is day 6 post-op. Slept well last night. Still on 4-hourly obs(observation). BP：160 over 100 in the morning. Had morning anti-hypertensive already. Dry dressing intact with no ooze from the drain site. On a light diet and bowels opened last night. Needs to be reviewed by his doctor. Oral Keflex QID (quarter in die,每日 4 次) 12：00 midday.

Exercise

Please fill in a handover report according to the information given below.

【20 床，王洪，男，50 岁，主治医生为王大林。左腿膝盖以上截肢，患者有非胰岛素依赖型糖尿病（NIDDM），需控制饮食。每日 4 次观察生命体征及血糖值（BSL）随机排查。敷料和绷带完整，行动需轮椅。】

Extended Knowledge

I. First Aid—Broken Hand Treatment

Step 1 Stop bleeding if necessary.

1. Apply firm pressure with a clean cloth until bleeding stops.

2. If the bone is pushing through the skin, do not touch it or try to put it back in place.

Step 2 Control swelling.

1. Apply an ice pack (do not put ice directly against the skin).

2. If possible, remove any jewelry immediately.

Step 3 Immobilize the hand.

If the person's hand is numb or cold or the skin under the fingernails is blue, do not move the hand or arm. Otherwise:

1. Have the person bend the arm at the elbow.

2. Do not try to straighten the hand if it bent or deformed.

3. Tie a splint on the lower arm with fabric or elastic bandages. Cardboard, rolled-up newspaper or other stiff material can be used as a splint.

Step 4 See a health care provider immediately.

II. Knowledge Links

Communicating Effectively with Elderly Surgical Patients

A nurse's accepting attitude toward elderly surgical patients is an essential component of quality preoperative care. To reflect an accepting attitude toward aged patients, preoperative nurses are advised to examine their own attitudes and behaviors, recognize their stereotypical feelings, and be aware of their body language.

Body language reflects a person's innermost feelings: true attitudes show through body movements. To enhance communication with elderly patients and to show a caring, concerned attitude, apply the following behaviors.

• Maintain eye contact at eye level with the patient to show concern and interest. Most cultures place great value on maintaining eye contact during interactions. However, when you are using this nonverbal behavior, cultural differences should be considered. One group that sometimes finds prolonged eye contact unacceptable is native Americans. In addition, some cultures believe that a person's soul can be stolen through prolonged eye contact.

• Stand naturally. Do not slouch or cross your arms: these postures imply disinterest and may cause the patients to withdraw.

• Face the patient squarely. Turning away implies rejection and lack of interest.

• In a nonthreatening manner, gently touch the patient on the arm or shoulder. This communicates the desire to be helpful.

Touch usually is welcomed by elderly patients who often are missing touch in their lives. The way a patient responds, however, may depend on the culture origin. In some cultures, touch may imply

Note

63

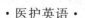

·医护英语·

扫码看
答案

something other than compassion. Most gerontologist researchers believe, however, that elderly patients are touched too little by nurses. Although cultural differences should be considered when determining appropriate touch, most researchers suggest that when caring for the elderly, some amount of touch generally is appropriate.

Note

Unit 9 Obstetrics and Pediatrics

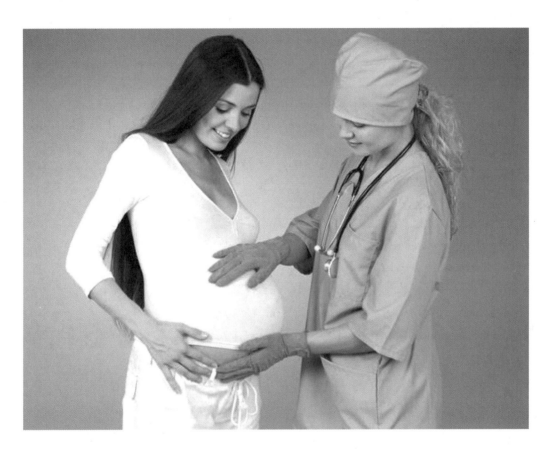

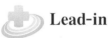 **Lead-in**

It is mother who brings a new baby to this world. They are the patients you will attend in this unit. To some degree, they are the most vulnerable group that needs your extreme patience and kindness. The part of obstetrics deals with the birth of children and the care of women before, during and after they give birth to children. Nurses play an integral and unquestionably important role during this time in a woman's life.

The part of pediatrics focuses on the care of infants and children. Because the patients are so young, nurses often form strong relational-ties with them in different ways by playing games with them, being goofy, or holding their hand during tough procedures.

Communication skills are needed while you deal with them.

Thinking & Talking

1. As a nurse, how do you help a mother deliver a baby smoothly?
2. As a nurse, how do you calm down a crying baby?

Note

Focus Listening

Conversation 1

扫码听
对话1

Directions：*This is a conversation between Linda and a nurse. The nurse is examining Linda, a first-time mother, who is having labor pains. Listen carefully and decide whether the following statements are true (T) or false (F).*

( ) 1. Relaxation helps the patient feel less labor pain.

( ) 2. To check the patient's pulse, blood pressure and temperature, the nurse asks the patient to lie still.

( ) 3. The nurse places a pillow under the patient to ease her labor pain.

( ) 4. When the labor pain gets stronger, the patient is recommended to take a deep breath regularly.

New Words & Expressions

扫码听
单词

labor [ˈleɪbə(r)]	n. 分娩
contraction [kənˈtrækʃən]	n. 子宫收缩
distract [dɪˈstrækt]	v. 转移,使分心
hip [hɪp]	n. 臀部
massage [ˈmæsɑːʒ]	n. 按摩,推拿
rhythmically [ˈrɪðmɪklɪ]	adv. 有节奏地
moan [məʊn]	v. 抱怨,呻吟
endure [ɪnˈdjʊə(r)]	v. 忍耐,容忍

Conversation 2

扫码听
对话2

Directions：*You will hear a conversation among a doctor, Tom and Tom's mother. The doctor is in the pediatric consulting room. She is having a conversation with the patient, Tom and his mother. Listen carefully and fill in the blanks according to the conversation.*

Tom has a temperature, headache, 1._____ and rash. After checking, the nurse says he has 2._____ and red tonsils, red 3._____ and 4._____ all over his body. So he must have a 5._____ test. It shows that his white blood count is 6._____. He is probably having a 7._____, which is a kind of 8._____ disease. To protect people around him and ensure a quick recovery, he has to stay by himself and eat 9._____ and drink 10._____.

New Words & Expressions

Note

rash [ræʃ]	n. 皮疹
fever [ˈfiːvə(r)]	n. 发烧,发热;狂热
sticker [ˈstɪkə(r)]	n. 粘贴标签
tonsil [ˈtɒnsɪl]	n. 扁桃体,扁桃腺

scared [skeəd]   adj. 害怕的

infectious [ɪn'fekʃəs]   adj. 传染的，传染性的

digestible [daɪ'dʒestəbl]   adj. 易消化的

penicillin [ˌpenɪ'sɪlɪn]   n. 盘尼西林（青霉素）

injection [ɪn'dʒekʃən]   n. 注射，注射剂

scarlet fever   猩红热

扫码听
单词

Group Discussion & Role Playing

1. Discuss with your partner. Change the patient types or demands and redesign the conversation.

2. Display the conversation you've made.

3. After one group finishes the performance，others make comments.

Intensive Reading

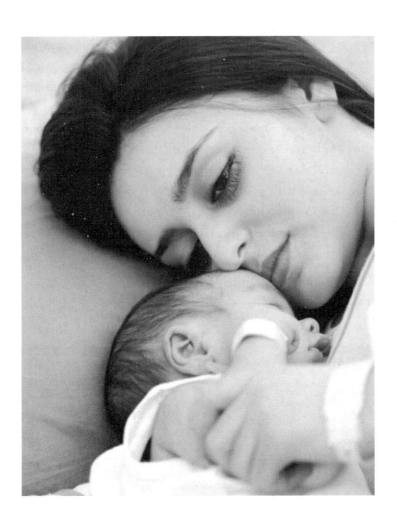

扫码听
课文

Note

Postpartum Recovery

The moment you give birth to a baby, you are officially a mother. Every new mother experiences the first few hours after giving birth a little differently, but there are some common elements.

In the early days, new mothers are not used to the frequency of infant nursing, but this is a healthy response from your newborn for both them and you. Frequent breastfeeding helps stimulate oxytocin, contract and shrink uterus. These uterus contractions are called postpartum afterpains. Some women feel them, especially during breastfeeding, while others don't. Meanwhile, this shrinking helps make the placental insertion point smaller so that you hopefully lose less blood.

If you've had a vaginal birth, you will be sore and swollen from giving birth. The generous use of a peri bottle makes going to the bathroom easier. Fill the peri bottle with body temperature water and use it to rinse the perineal area rather than wiping. This is especially helpful if you have any tearing or stitches.

If you have delivered by a cesarean section, you may not have vaginal pain and swelling. However, you have to be very careful with your incision, like moving carefully, protecting it when breastfeeding, even avoiding stairs or things that put strain on the incision. As nursing after a cesarean section is relatively challenging, it is useful to know some tips for breastfeeding after cesarean.

No matter how you gave birth, no matter how easy your delivery was, the first six weeks postpartum are considered a "recovery" period. Your body needs a chance to regroup, so take time to rest and be gentle with yourself.

For many women, lochia can last for about six weeks postpartum. During this period, there are visible signs of recovery like blood loss and loose skin, your body is recovering internally too. The incision from a cesarean takes many weeks to mend. Tearing or episiotomy from a vaginal birth also takes time to fully heal. The tissues themselves through which the baby has passed also take time to return to a state more similar to that experienced prior to birth.

Some women feel like their body and organs do fully return to their pre-baby state, while others never feel 100% the same as they did before childbirth.

Every new mother, regardless of delivery method, please keep in mind that the weeks after giving birth should be a time of patience with yourself. Your life is different now. A new baby needs to be nursed frequently. This helps them to grow. Thus, you are supposed to sit, be still, and let your body recover. Be patient with this process. It may feel as though you are getting nothing done, but recovering from the major event of childbirth and breastfeeding a baby are big jobs which take time, effort, and focus.

New Words & Expressions

postpartum [pəʊst'pɑːtəm]	adj. 产后的
frequency ['friːkwənsɪ]	n. 频率,频繁
infant ['ɪnfənt]	n. 婴儿,幼儿
breastfeeding ['brestˌfiːdɪŋ]	n. 母乳哺育
stimulate ['stɪmjʊleɪt]	v. 刺激;鼓舞,激励
oxytocin [ˌɒksɪ'təʊsɪn]	n. 催产素,缩宫素
uterus ['juːtərəs]	n. 子宫

placental [plə'sentəl]	adj. 胎盘的,胎座的
insertion [ɪn'sɜːʃən]	n. 插入,嵌入
afterpains ['ɑːftəpeɪnz]	n. 产后痛
vaginal [və'dʒaɪnəl]	adj. 阴道的
peri bottle	冲洗罐
rinse [rɪns]	v. 漱,冲洗掉
perineal [peri'niːəl]	adj. 会阴的
tear [tɪə(r)]	v. 撕裂,撕破
stitch [stɪtʃ]	n. 缝线,(缝纫的)一针
cesarean [sɪ'zeərɪən]	adj. 剖腹产的
strain [streɪn]	n. 担忧,压力
delivery [dɪ'lɪvərɪ]	n. 分娩,递送
lochia ['lɒkɪə]	n. 恶露,产褥排泄物
internally [ɪn'tɜːnəlɪ]	adv. 内部地,国内地
episiotomy [ɪˌpiːsɪ'ɒtəmɪ]	n. 会阴切开术
tissue ['tɪʃjuː]	n. (人、动植物细胞的)组织

Exercises

Exercise 1. Decide whether the following statements are true (T) or false (F) according to the text.

( ) 1. Frequent breastfeeding is beneficial for both mother and the newborn.

( ) 2. The occurrence of postpartum afterpains vary from person to person.

( ) 3. It is recommended to wipe the perineal area rather than rinse in the first few days postpartum.

( ) 4. Breastfeeding after a cesarean is challenging.

( ) 5. All women can return to their pre-baby state after about six weeks postpartum.

Exercise 2. Fill in the blanks with the words given below, changing the form if necessary.

infant	stimulate	element	insertion
delivery	tissue	contract	frequency

1. Many women will tell you that the breathing techniques can be absolutely useless during labor and _____ .

2. When milk teeth are trying to push their way through, the _____ will become very excited.

3. The government will announce new measures to _____ the property market within a week.

4. Spending a great deal of time out in the sun may damage the skin and _____ beneath.

5. The front leg quadriceps (四头肌)_____ to support the body weight.

Exercise 3. Translate the following Chinese sentences into English.

1. 母乳喂养帮助子宫收缩。

2. 不管分娩过程多快,产后都需要长时间恢复。

3. 95%的初产妇在分娩过程中会经历阴道撕裂。

4. 有些女性觉得自己的身体和器官能完全恢复到产前。

5. 剖腹产的女性需要更多的时间恢复。

Note

Learning More

Ⅰ. Affixes & Roots of Medical Terms

Affixes & Roots	Chinese	More Words
peri-	周围,近	perianal 肛周的;periadenitis 腺周炎
-tomy	切除术	lobotomy 脑叶切除术;appendicectomy 阑尾切除术

Match the English expressions with the right Chinese phrases.

1. periacinal
2. appendicectomy
3. cardiotomy
4. cervicotomy

A. 心脏切开术
B. 腺泡周的
C. 子宫颈切开术
D. 阑尾切除术

Ⅱ. Vocabulary Expansion

Match the Chinese phrases with the right English expressions.

A. diaper	B. cramp	C. primipara
D. dehydration	E. dilate	F. pubic
G. antibiotics	H. fetal	I. womb
J. vaccinate	K. nipple	L. pregnancy

1. (　　)抗生素　　　　(　　)扩张
2. (　　)子宫　　　　　(　　)初产妇
3. (　　)接种疫苗　　　(　　)脱水
4. (　　)尿布　　　　　(　　)阴部的
5. (　　)乳头　　　　　(　　)胎儿的

Practical Writing

Birth Certificate(出生证明)

出生证明是证明新生儿身份的一份重要文件,通常包括以下内容:婴儿的性别、出生时间、出生地点、父母的姓名、身高、体重。

Sample

<table>
<tr><td colspan="2" align="center">**Birth Certificate**</td></tr>
<tr><td colspan="2">This is to certify that Ding Yi (female) was born on April 6, 2011 in Shanghai, China, to Ding Fang, father and Yi Yang, mother. Weight:3.0 kg. Height:49 cm.
International Peace Maternity and Child Health Hospital</td></tr>
<tr><td colspan="2" align="right">(sealed)
Signature
(sealed)
Date:April 11, 2011</td></tr>
</table>

Exercise

Please write a Birth Certificate according to the information given below.

姓名:王天一　性别:男　体重:3.5 kg　身高:50 cm

出生日期:2015 年 8 月 2 日

出生地:上海第五人民医院

父亲姓名:王林　母亲姓名:周新新

Extended Knowledge

Ⅰ. First Aid—Choking babies less than 1-year-old

Step 1 Assessing the situation.

1. Allow the baby to cough. If the baby is coughing or gagging, this means that his or her airway is only partially blocked.

2. Look for symptoms of choking. If the baby is unable to cry or make noise, his or her airway is completely blocked.

Step 2 Call for emergency medical support.

Step 3 Position the baby correctly.

1. Lay the baby on his or her back along the length of your forearm.

2. Make a baby sandwich by placing your other arm over the baby's front. Hold the jaw between your thumb and fingers.

3. Flip the infant in your arms, so he or she is now facing downward and resting on the forearm of the arm that was originally on top.

4. Rest the arm with the baby in it on your leg. To proceed, the baby's head should not be higher that his or her chest.

Step 4 Begin five back blows.

Use the base of your palm to apply 5 blows to the infant's back, right at the area between the shoulder blades. You should do this with a decent amount of force.

Step 5 Change the baby's position to begin chest compressions.

1. Turn the baby back over, so he or she is facing upward again. Use othe sandwich method described above. Make sure that your bottom hand is supporting the baby's head.

Note

2. Rest your arm and the baby on your leg again, keeping his or her head lower than the chest.

Step 6 Apply chest compressions.

1. Place two or three fingertips in the center of the baby's chest, just below their nipples.

2. Give 5 firm compressions on the chest. The right amount of pressure causes the breastbone to give about 1/2 to 1 inch and then retaliate between compressions.

Step 7 Repeat front compressions and back thrusts until the child coughs, breathes or falls unconscious.

Warning: Do not attempt to remove the obstruction by hand.

Ⅱ. Knowledge Links

Baby Blues vs. Postpartum Depression

It's normal to have the baby blues during the postpartum period. This typically happens a few days after giving birth and can last for up to two weeks. In most cases, you won't be experiencing symptoms all the time, and your symptoms will vary. About 70 to 80 percent of new mothers experience mood swings or negative feelings after giving birth. Baby blues caused by hormonal changes and symptoms may include: unexplained crying, irritability, insomnia, sadness, mood changes, restlessness.

The baby blues are different from postpartum depression. Postpartum depression occurs when symptoms last for more than two weeks.

Additional symptoms may include feelings of guilt and worthlessness, and loss of interest in daily activities. Some women with postpartum depression withdraw from their family, have no interest in their baby, and have thoughts of hurting their baby.

Postpartum depression requires medical treatment. Speak with your doctor if you have depression that lasts longer than two weeks after giving birth, or if you have thoughts of harming your baby. Postpartum depression can develop at any time after giving birth, even up to a year after delivery.

扫码看
答案

Unit 10   Traditional Chinese Medicine

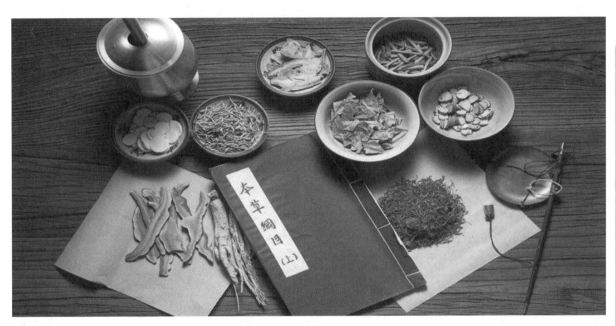

扫码看
PPT

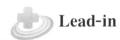 **Lead-in**

Traditional Chinese medicine (TCM) has been passed on for thousands of years in China. Even in European and American countries where western medicines are popular, more and more people recognize the magical effects of TCM. Generally speaking, the therapeutic methods of TCM are divided into two categories: drug therapy and non-drug therapy.

Drug therapy is also named as TCM herbal treatment. Through the internal and external use of Chinese herbal medicine, it can directly act on the inside and outside of the human body. Strengthening the body and eliminating pathogens, regulating the balance of Yin and Yang, and increasing the immune function of the body.

Non-drug therapies include traditional Chinese acupuncture, cupping, Guasha, acupoint application and other methods, which help to regulate the normal operation of Zang Fu organs, meridians, Qi and blood, so as to achieve the effect of treating and preventing diseases.

Thinking & Talking

1. Please list names of some Chinese herbs that you know.

2. What other non-drug therapies do you know?

Note

Focus Listening

Conversation 1

扫码听
对话1

Directions：*You will hear a conversation between Ms. Li and a doctor. Ms. Li has been sneezing, nose stuffing and itching recently. She comes to the TCM for help. Listen to the conversation carefully and choose the best answer for each of the following questions.*

1. Does Ms. Li feel itchy in the eyes? _____.
A. Yes, she does B. No, she doesn't C. It's not mentioned

2. Which department does the doctor advise Ms. Li to go first? _____.
A. Emergency B. Surgery C. Allergy

3. What disease has NOT been mentioned in this conversation? _____.
A. Bronchitis B. Skin disorder C. Allergic rhinitis

4. Can children receive dog day moxibustion treatment? _____.
A. Yes, they can B. No, they can't C. It's not mentioned

5. How many times should the patients have the plasters? _____.
A. Two B. Three C. Four

New Words & Expressions

扫码听
单词

itch ['ɪtʃ]	n. 痒
allergic rhinitis [ə'lɜːdʒɪk raɪ'naɪtɪs]	过敏性鼻炎
allergy ['ælədʒɪ]	n. 过敏反应
desensitization [diːˌsensətaɪ'zeɪʃən]	n. 脱敏
immunotherapy [ˌɪmjʊnəʊ'θerəpɪ]	n. 免疫疗法
dog day moxibustion treatment	三伏药物敷贴疗法
acupoint ['ækjʊpɒɪnt]	n. 穴位
asthma ['æsmə]	n. 哮喘，气喘
bronchitis [brɒŋ'kaɪtɪs]	n. 支气管炎
rheumatic [ru'mætɪk]	n. 风湿病；adj. 风湿病的

Conversation 2

扫码听
对话2

Directions：*You will hear a conversation between Ms. Wang and a doctor. Ms. Wang has been losing her sleep and appetite. She comes to the TCM department for help. Listen carefully and fill in the blanks according to the conversation.*

（A：Doctor B：Ms. Wang）

A：Hello, please have a seat.

B：I've been losing my sleep and my appetite.

A：How long have you been like this?

B：About 1. _____ months. It really tortures me a lot.

A：Are there any other discomforts?

Note

B：2. _____ , and sometimes dizziness.

A：Have you taken any medicine?

B：Yes. I've been taking 3. _____ medicines these days，but I am also worried about their 4. _____ , so I want to try Chinese herbal medicine.

A：All right. Please give me your hand and I'll take your pulse.

(*during pulse diagnosis...*)

A：You have wiry and rapid 5. _____ . Are you in a bad mood recently? Do you always get angry?

B：Yes.

A：Do you have 6. _____ taste in your mouth?

B：Yes.

A：Let me have a look at your tongue，please.

(*Pulse examination is completed.*)

A：You have red tongue with yellow coating. According to your symptoms，this is caused by stagnated liver-Qi changing into fire. You need to disperse stagnated liver-Qi，eliminate heat，and calm the mind. I'll give you some Chinese herbs for 7. _____ use. In addition，you also need acupuncture. Internal and external conditioning can recover your body gradually.

B：All right.

A：This is your prescription. Please get the herbs at the 8. _____ . They can help you to decoct the herbs into patent medicine if you like. This is your acupuncture schedule.

B：Thank you very much.

A：You're welcome.

New Words & Expressions

appetite ['æpɪtaɪt]	n. 食欲，嗜好
side effect	副作用
stagnate [stæg'neɪt]	v. 停滞，淤塞
disperse [dɪ'spɜːs]	v. 分散，使散开
acupuncture ['ækjʊˌpʌŋktʃə(r)]	n. 针灸
recover [rɪ'kʌvə(r)]	v. 恢复
decoct [dɪ'kɒkt]	v. 煎，熬
patent medicine	成药

扫码听
单词

Group Discussion & Role Playing

1. Discuss with your partner. Change the patient types or demands and redesign the conversation.

2. Display the conversation you've made.

3. After one group finishes the performance，others make comments.

Note

75

Intensive Reading

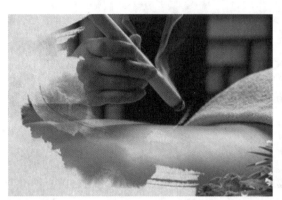
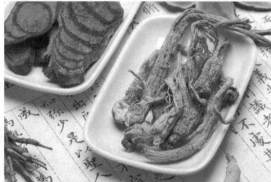

Traditional Chinese Medicine

In the view of traditional Chinese medicine, we live in a universe in which everything is interconnected. The human body has inseparable relations with the external nature. Even the human body itself is an organic whole. The mind and the body are not viewed separately. What happens to one part of the body affects every other part of the body.

According to ancient Chinese philosophy, human beings and other forms of life on earth are the product of Qi, which is a vital force or energy to control the working and functioning of the human mind and the body. Only when Qi and blood, Yin and Yang as well as man and nature are in harmony can the health of human beings be ensured. Otherwise, if the balance is broken, one will be attacked by illness.

In order to promote smooth circulation of Qi and blood, maintain fitness, help prevent diseases and ensure quick recovery, TCM includes a variety of traditional Chinese therapies, such as herbal medicine; acupuncture, moxibustion, point plaster application, cupping, Tuina and Guasha; changing diet and lifestyle; and exercising (often in the form of Qigong or Taichi).

The practice of acupuncture is based on the theories of meridians and acupuncture points. It is the insertion of very fine needles into acupuncture points just beneath the body surface in order to relieve pain, treat illness and promote health.

Traditional Chinese medicine regards the dog days of summer and the coldest days of winter as the switch points of Yin and Yang. People rush to hospitals to apply a medicated plaster to the acupuncture points to prevent respiratory diseases, allergic disorders, rheumatic diseases and obstinate skin disorders.

Although the principles of traditional Chinese medicine may be difficult for some to understand, more and more people worldwide begin to study and practice TCM. The reasons for the increasing interest are due to its excellent therapeutic effects and mild toxic and side effects. Traditional Chinese medicine is a great treasure of Chinese culture and of the world culture as well.

New Words & Expressions

vital force	生机,生命力
circulation [ˌsɜːkjʊˈleɪʃən]	n. 流通,传播

therapy [ˈθerəpɪ]	n. 治疗，疗法
moxibustion [ˌmɒksɪˈbʌstʃən]	n. 艾灸，中医灸法
plaster [ˈplɑːstə(r)]	n. 石膏，膏药
meridian [məˈrɪdɪən]	n. 经络
medicated [ˈmedɪkeɪtɪd]	adj. 药物的，含药的
obstinate [ˈɒbstɪnət]	adj. 顽固的，倔强的
toxic [ˈtɒksɪk]	adj. 有毒的，中毒的

扫码听
单词

Exercises

Exercise 1. Decide whether the following statements are true (T) or false (F) according to the text.

(   ) 1. The human body is an organic whole. It has no relationship with the nature.

(   ) 2. People would be unhealthy if the balance of Qi and blood be interrupted.

(   ) 3. Acupuncturists insert needles into acupoints according to the theory of Yin-Yang.

(   ) 4. The dog day moxibustion treatment is helpful to treat asthma, allergic rhinitis and skin disorders.

(   ) 5. Many people would like to use TCM because of its negative side effects.

Exercise 2. Fill in the blanks with the words given below, changing the form if necessary.

| side effects | conditioning | appetite | moxibustion |
| respiratory | immunotherapy | toxic | pulse |

1. _____ diseases are common diseases in winter.

2. _____ is used as a supplement during the performance of acupuncture.

3. Internal and external _____ can make the body recover quickly.

4. The four TCM methods of diagnosis are observation, listening, questioning, and _____-taking.

5. The treatment for allergic rhinitis is _____.

Exercise 3. Translate the following Chinese sentences into English.

1. 我最近总是失眠，而且食欲不振。
2. 许多人喜欢使用中药是因为中药副作用小。
3. 定期运动有助于促进气血循环。
4. 非药物疗法包括针灸、推拿和拔罐。
5. 中医认为，人体与自然密切相关。

Learning More

Ⅰ. Affixes & Roots of Medical Terms

Affixes & Roots	Chinese	More Words
allerg(o)-	过敏	allergen 过敏原；allergy 过敏性反应
immun(o)-	免疫	immunity 免疫力；immunotherapy 免疫疗法
acu-	针，尖锐	acupuncture 针灸；acupressure 指针疗法

Note

Affixes & Roots	Chinese	More Words
bronch(i)-	支气管	bronchitis 支气管炎；bronchiectasis 支气管扩张
rhin(o)-	鼻	rhinitis 鼻炎；rhinobyon 鼻塞
rheumat(o)-	风湿	rheumatic 风湿病；rheumatology 风湿病学
pharmac(o)-	药，药学	pharmacy 药房；pharmacist 药剂师
-therapy	疗法	immunotherapy 免疫疗法；physiotherapy 物理疗法

Match the English expressions with the right Chinese phrases.

1. rhinitis   A. 风湿病学

2. acupuncture   B. 过敏原

3. rheumatology   C. 鼻炎

4. bronchiectasis   D. 针灸

5. allergen   E. 免疫疗法

6. immunotherapy   F. 支气管扩张

Ⅱ. Vocabulary Expansion

Match the Chinese phrases with the right English expressions.

A. pulse	B. acupuncture	C. patent medicine
D. moxibustion	E. asthma	F. appetite
G. allergic rhinitis	H. dog days	I. side effect
J. meridians	K. Chinese herbal medicine	L. acupoint

1.（   ）食欲   （   ）中草药

2.（   ）脉搏   （   ）副作用

3.（   ）穴位   （   ）哮喘

4.（   ）针灸   （   ）过敏性鼻炎

5.（   ）经络   （   ）艾灸

Practical Writing

Doctor's Certificate(诊断证明书)

医生的诊断证明书应该包含以下内容。

1. 诊断证明书的标题和开具日期。

2. 患者的基本信息，如姓名、性别、年龄。

3. 患者的入院时间、入院原因、治疗方式和治疗时间。

4. 出院时间、出院后的注意事项、建议休息时间。

5. 如果有必要，还要注明复查时间。

6. 医生签字。

Sample

Doctor's Certificate

Oct. 20, 2019

This is to certify that the patient, Mr. Mike Johnson, male, aged 40, was admitted into our hospital on October 10, 2019 for severe asthma. After emergency handling and eleven days of treatment, he has got well and can be discharged on October 20, 2019. It is suggested that he do not do any physical exercises and take a good rest for one week at home before going back to his work.

Jane White

Chief Physician

(signature)

Exercise

Please write a doctor's certificate according to the information given below.

【李明,男,19 岁,2019 年 8 月 6 日因肺炎住院,经过 1 周的治疗已经痊愈,并将于 2019 年 8 月 12 日出院。建议出院后再休息 3 天。如果再次出现发热症状,须及时就医。】

Extended Knowledge

Ⅰ. First Aid—Choking Adults

Step 1 Assess the situation.

1. Make sure the person is choking and determine whether it is a partial or total airway obstruction.

2. If a person is experiencing mild choking, or partial airway obstruction, you are better off letting him/her cough to remove the obstruction himself. Do not use back blows.

Step 2 Administer firstaid.

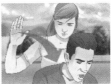

If the person is choking severely or suffering from a total airway obstruction and is conscious, communicate your intent to perform first aid.

Step 3 Give back blows.

1. Stand behind the person and slightly off to one side.

2. Support the person's chest with one hand and lean the person forward.

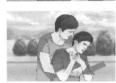

3. Administer up to five forceful blows between the person's shoulder blades with the heel of your hand (between your palm and wrist).

4. Pause after each blow to see if the blockage has cleared.

If not, give up to five abdominal thrusts.

Step 4 Administer abdominal thrusts (Heimlich maneuver).

1. Stand behind the choking victim and wrap your arms around his/her waist.

2. Make a fist with one hand and hold the fist with the other hand.

3. Place the thumb-side of your fist right above the victim's navel.

4. Lean the victim slightly forward and press into his/her abdomen with a hard, upward thrust.

5. Do this thrusting action up to five times. Check after each thrust to see if the blockage is gone.

Note

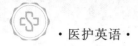

Stop if the victim loses consciousness.

Ⅱ. Knowledge Links

Acupressure

Acupressure is an ancient art of healing believed by some people to be even older than acupuncture. It involves the use of the fingers (and in some cases, the toes) to press key points on the surface of the skin to stimulate the body's natural ability to heal itself. Pressing on these points relieves muscle tension, which promotes the circulation of blood and Qi to aid in the healing process.

What's the difference between acupressure and acupuncture?

Acupressure and acupuncture are actually quite alike. In fact, acupressure is sometimes referred to as "needleless acupuncture", because both forms of healing use the same points to achieve the desired results. The main difference between the two treatments is that an acupuncturist stimulates points by inserting needles, whereas an acupressurist stimulates the same points using finger pressure.

扫码看
答案

Note

Unit 11　Rehabilitation

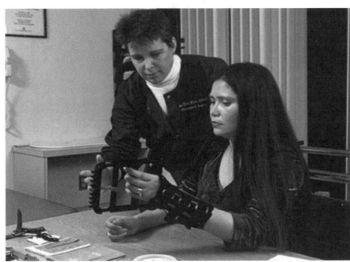

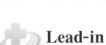 **Lead-in**

Rehabilitation includes a wide range of activities in addition to medical care, including physical, psychosocial and occupational therapies. In other words, rehabilitation is defined as an educational, problem-solving process that focuses on activity limitations and aims to optimize patients' social participation and well-being, so as to reduce stress on families. Rehabilitation serves as two objectives. One is the rehabilitation of individuals. The other is educating all health care professionals, as well as the general public. If the objectives are achieved, we will see a new society in which people with disabilities have a fair chance to work, enjoy life, and live as independently as possible. Thus, a central focus of rehabilitation is the quality of life.

Thinking & Talking

1. What is the definition of rehabilitation?
2. What are the objectives of rehabilitation?

Focus Listening

Conversation 1

Directions: *You will hear a conversation between Mrs. Smith and a nurse. The nurse comes to*

 Note

扫码听
对话 1

inform Mrs. Smith of the performance of tube feeding. Listen carefully and decide whether the following statements are true（T）or false（F）.

（　　）1. Mrs. Smith was watching TV when the nurse came in.

（　　）2. Mrs. Smith was happy when she was told to have a tube put through her nose into her stomach.

（　　）3. The nurse promised to stop feeding the tube if Mrs. Smith wanted a break.

（　　）4. The nurse got the permission from Mrs. Smith to feed the tube.

New Words & Expressions

扫码听
单词

tube [tjuːb]	n. 管子
comfortable ['kʌmftəbl]	adj. 舒服的
nutrition [njuː'trɪʃən]	n. 营养,养分
unbearable [ʌn'beərəbl]	adj. 难以忍受的
swallow ['swɒləʊ]	v. 吞咽
uneasy [ʌn'iːzɪ]	adj. 不舒服的,不安的
kill time	消磨时间
tend to	倾向于,趋向
mark my words	记住我的话

Conversation 2

扫码听
对话 2

Directions：*You will hear a conversation between* <u>Mr. Silverman</u> *and* <u>a nurse</u>. *The nurse comes to instruct Mr. Silverman how to manage to take a bath by himself. Arrange the following steps in a proper sequence based on the conversation.*

1. Slide along the transfer board onto the stool which is in the bathtub.

2. Have the wheelchair fixed against the bathtub's side.

3. Lift your legs and put them into the bathtub with the help of the hands.

4. Put the stool into the bathtub.

5. Place one end of the transfer board on your wheelchair and the other on the stool.

The correct order is _____.

New Words & Expressions

扫码听
单词

stinky ['stɪŋkɪ]	adj. 发臭的,令人厌恶的
bathtub ['bɑːθtʌb]	n. 浴缸
transfer [træns'fɜː(r)]	n. 转移
manage ['mænɪdʒ]	v. 完成,管理
slide [slaɪd]	v. 滑行
bottom ['bɒtəm]	n. 底部,屁股
not sleep a wink	完全没睡觉
function as	起着……作用

Note

Group Discussion & Role Playing

1. Discuss with your partner. Change the patient types or demands and redesign the conversation.

2. Display the conversation you've made.

3. After one group finishes the performance, others make comments.

Intensive Reading

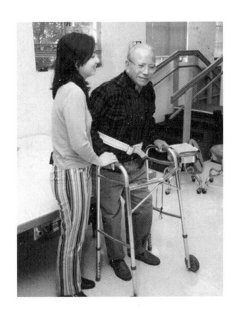

扫码听
课文

The Rehabilitation Team

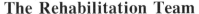

The rehabilitation team typically includes physician, nurse, social worker, physical therapist and occupational therapist. Other subjects, such as speech pathology, clinical psychology, pharmacology, or nutrition, may be requested for consultation as needed.

Physicians

A physician who specializes in rehabilitative medicine is called a physiatrist. Most inpatient rehabilitation departments employ physiatrists. A primary care physician may also supervise the patient's medical problems.

Nurses

Nursing staff members assess the patient at the beginning, carry out the rehabilitation plan, observe the process of treatment, and record the progress of the patient. They cooperate with the team and make sure that the patient with other medical problems get appropriate care. The nurse emphasizes the goals and techniques of therapy, provides education for the patient and the family, and is responsible for ensuring continuity of care.

Physical Therapists (PTs)

Physical therapists come to help the patient achieve self-management by focusing on gross motor

Note

83

skills. For instance, PTs teach clients how to use crutches, prostheses and wheelchairs for mobility. They may also teach the way to perform certain activities of daily livings (ADLs), such as transferring into or out of bed, ambulating and toileting. Moreover, PTs use hot or cold compresses, ultrasound, or electrical stimulation to relieve pain, reduce swelling, and improve muscle tone.

Occupational Therapists (OTs)

Occupational therapists work to develop the patient's fine motor skills used for ADLs, such as those required for eating, hygiene and dressing. OTs also teach patients how to perform independent living skills, such as cooking and shopping. Many inpatient rehabilitation facilities have fully furnished and equipped apartments where patients can practice independent living skills in a mock setting under supervision. To accomplish these outcomes, OTs teach skills related to coordination (e. g., hand movements) and cognitive retraining.

Speech-Language Pathologists (SLPs)

Speech-language pathologists (SLPs) evaluate and retrain patients with speech, language, or swallowing problems. Some patients, especially those who have experienced a head injury or stroke, have difficulty with both speech and language. Those who have had a stroke also may have dysphagia. SLPs provide screening and testing for dysphagia. If the patient has this problem, the SLP recommends appropriate foods and feeding techniques.

New Words & Expressions

rehabilitation [ˌriːhəˌbɪlɪˈteɪʃən]	n. 康复
physician [fɪˈzɪʃən]	n. 医生,内科医生
psychology [saɪˈkɒlədʒɪ]	n. 心理学
pharmacology [ˌfɑːməˈkɒlədʒɪ]	n. 药物学,药理学
rehabilitative [riːhəˈbɪlɪtətɪv]	adj. 康复的,复原的
physiatrist [ˌfɪzɪˈætrɪst]	n. 理疗师
assess [əˈses]	v. 评定,估价
gross [ɡrəʊs]	adj. 粗略的,总共的
prostheses [prɒsˈθiːsiːz]	假体(如假肢、假眼或假牙等)(prosthesis 的名词复数)
ambulate [ˈæmbjʊleɪt]	v. 走动,步行
compress [kəmˈpres]	n. 敷布,压布
mock [mɒk]	adj. 模拟的
coordination [kəʊˌɔːdɪˈneɪʃn]	n. 协调,调和
cognitive [ˈkɒɡnɪtɪv]	adj. 认知的,认识的
pathologist [pəˈθɒlədʒɪst]	n. 病理学家
dysphagia [dɪsˈfeɪdʒɪə]	n. 吞咽困难
screening [ˈskriːnɪŋ]	n. 筛选
physical therapist	物理治疗师
occupational therapist	作业治疗师
electrical stimulation	电刺激治疗
muscle tone	肌张力,肌肉紧张度
fine motor skills	精细运动技能

扫码听
单词

Note

84

Exercises

Exercise 1. Decide whether the following statements are true (T) or false (F) according to the text.

(　　) 1. The rehabilitation team typically includes physicians, nurses, social workers, speech-language pathologists, and occupational therapists.

(　　) 2. A physician who specializes in rehabilitative medicine is called a physiatrist.

(　　) 3. The nurse reinforces the goals and techniques of therapy, provides education, and is responsible for ensuring continuity of care.

(　　) 4. Physical therapists come to help the patient achieve self-management by focusing on fine motor skills.

(　　) 5. Occupational therapists work to develop the patient's gross motor skills used for ADLs.

Exercise 2. Fill in the blanks with the words or phrases given below, changing the form if necessary.

clinical	assess	inpatient	rehabilitation
ambulate	physical therapist	hygiene	carry out

1. The old people with disabilities are using new equipment to do _____ exercises.

2. A nurse will phone those pregnant women for a 15-minute consultation and _____ the effect of health education.

3. The patient was allowed to _____ in the room.

4. A _____ may advise routine exercise to help the patient maintain joint mobility.

5. A clinic nurse's job is to first work out a plan, then _____ the plan, evaluate and get feedbacks.

Exercise 3. Translate the following Chinese sentences into English.

1. 我这段时间住院治疗的目标是什么？
2. 她的精细运动技能受到影响，所以每两周要看一次作业治疗师和物理治疗师。
3. 他们帮助患者洗澡、穿衣和保持个人卫生。
4. 糖尿病增加了患心脏病和脑卒中的危险。
5. 这些疾病早期很少或没有症状，并且也没有有效的筛查试验。

Learning More

Ⅰ. Affixes & Roots of Medical Terms

Affixes & Roots	Chinese	More Words
post-	后	postoperative 术后的；postpartum 产后的
dys-	异常	dysphagia 吞咽困难；dysplasia 发育不良
psych(o)-	精神，意志	psychiatry 精神病学；psychopathology 精神病理学
phag(o)-	吃，吞	dysphagia 吞咽困难；phagocyte 吞噬细胞
physic-	身体的；物理的	physician 医生；physiatrist 理疗师
path(o)-；-(o)pathy	疾病	pathologist 病理学家；neuropathy 神经病

Match the English expressions with the right Chinese phrases.

1. dysphagia   A. 术后的
2. postoperative   B. 医生
3. physician   C. 病理学家
4. pathologist   D. 吞咽困难

Ⅱ. Vocabulary Expansion

Match the Chinese phrases with the right English expressions.

A. tube	B. ultrasound	C. related to
D. nutrition	E. mobility	F. occupational therapist
G. swallow	H. hygiene	I. function as
J. relieve	K. stroke	L. transfer

1. (   )转移   (   )解除,减轻
2. (   )吞咽   (   )超声
3. (   )移动性   (   )与……有关
4. (   )卫生   (   )脑卒中
5. (   )作业治疗师   (   )管子

Practical Writing

Notice(通知)

通知通常分为两大类:口头通知和书面通知。通知(或布告)的格式和书信不相同,不写对方的地址和名称,也不一定用称呼和结束语。

医学上的通知多为书面通知。书面通知有一定的格式:上有标题"Notice(或 Announcement)",其后既可编号也可不编号;出通知(或布告)的单位名称,应写在"Notice"一词上面,也可写在正文右下角;较正式的通知(或布告)必须有单位负责人的署名,可写在正文的右下角,署名下面写上职务;发通知的日期,一般写在左下角或右上角,但有时也可以省略。

Sample

Shanghai Renji Hospital Notice of Critical Illness Claim Form
Patient:Tom Smith
DOB:Sep. 22,1954
Gender:male
Symptoms:sharp headache, vomiting and deep shock
Diagnosis:stroke
Treatment:cardiorespiratory resuscitation
<div align="right">Mar. 20,2020</div>

Note

续表

Dear Mr. Smith,

We are sorry to announce that your condition is becoming increasingly severe. We'd like you to understand that the hospital is committed to applying all effective treatments including cardiorespiratory resuscitation. Please inform your doctor immediately after receiving the notice if you should have any other requests.

Doctor John Smith

Geriatrics Department

Exercise

Please write a notice of critical illness claim form according to the information given below.

【李玲,女,59岁,因糖尿病并发症住院,经诊断患者有脑血管病变,肾衰竭和脑卒中症状。目前症状非常危险,需要告知患者及家属除了控制血糖治疗外还需要进入重症监护室严密监测。】

Extended Knowledge

Ⅰ. First Aid—Adult Epilepsy

Step 1 Identify if a person has epilepsy.

The person has collapsed and is making sudden jerking movements. He/she may also have froth around his/her mouth. You may also find some form of identification on the person, such as a card, bracelet or necklace that gives information about his/her condition. If you can't find anything and are unsure if he/she has previously had seizures, call 120.

Step 2 Make the person safe and prevent injury.

Use a blanket or clothing to protect the person's head. Do not restrain the person. Restraining the person may cause injury to you or the person. Let the seizure run its normal course. Remove objects that may injure the person while he/she is having the seizure.

Step 3 Make sure the person keep breathing.

After the seizure, help the person to rest on his/her side with his/her head tilted back. This will make sure he/she keeps breathing.

Step 4 Call 120 if necessary.

Ⅱ. Knowledge Links

History of Rehabilitation Nursing

The Association of Rehabilitation Nurses (ARN) was formed by Susan Novak in 1974 with support from Lutheran General Hospital, in Park Ridge, Illinois, at a time when rehabilitation nursing became recognized as a nursing specialty. By 1976, ARN was formally recognized as a specialty nursing organization by the American Nurses Association (ANA). As the needs for these specialty nurses grew, ARN developed the Certified Rehabilitation Registered Nurse (CRRN) certification in 1984, and has turned over administration of the certification to the Rehabilitation Nursing Certification Board (RNCB), an autonomous component of ARN. The CRRN program is accredited by the American Board of Nursing Specialties.

Note

扫码看
答案

Evolution of the Specialty

An interdisciplinary healthcare specialty, rehabilitation evolved as many 20th century wartime soldiers, young men for the most part, survived injury but faced serious disability. As a result, military hospitals established rehabilitation units that focused extensive efforts on returning these young men to society. Soon, rehabilitation units and hospitals sprang up around the country and the interdisciplinary specialty of rehabilitation gained importance.

Rehabilitation Nursing Foundation (RNF)

As healthcare technology advances, more people are surviving injuries and diseases that once would have been fatal. People experiencing chronic illness are living longer, and the need for rehabilitation services continues to expand.

Mission: The Rehabilitation Nursing Foundation is dedicated to advancing rehabilitation nursing practice by promoting, developing, and/or engaging in educational activities and scientific research to improve the quality of health care to individuals with a disability or chronic illness.

Note

Unit 12　Ophthalmology & Otorhinolaryngology

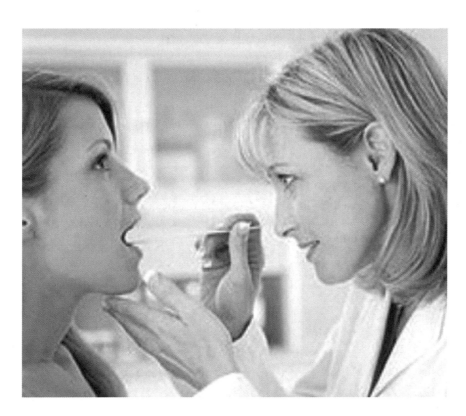

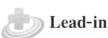 Lead-in

Ophthalmology is a branch of medicine concerned with people's eyes and the problems that affect them. And otolaryngology is the branch of medicine concerned with diagnosis and treatment of diseases of the ear, nose and throat. They are parts of the human body which are more susceptible to disease. Being the most troublesome parts of the body, they affect people's normal work and life. Without timely treatment, they are easy to cause various other diseases and the onsets of multiple complications. The eye, ear, nose and throat are distributed around the brain. Their small illnesses and small pains are often easily ignored by people. Meanwhile, they have developed gradually. As the saying goes, "A fire on the city wall brings disaster to the fish in the moat." The eye, ear, nose and throat are the most vulnerable to our brains. With the brain damaged, the whole body would be affected. The consequence could be disastrous.

Thinking & Talking

1. How to provide high-quality care for patients in Ophthalmology & Otolaryngology department?
2. Is humanistic care important for patients in Ophthalmology & Otolaryngology department?

Note

Focus Listening

Conversation 1

扫码听
对话 1

Directions: *This is a conversation between* <u>*Ms. Yang and a nurse*</u>. *Ms. Yang has got a pain and a purulent flow in her ear. She comes to the otolaryngology department for help. Listen carefully and decide whether the following statements are true（T）or false（F）.*

(　　) 1. Ms. Yang's hearing is not affected.

(　　) 2. There is a purulent flow in her ear.

(　　) 3. She does not feel any pain when the nurse presses on the mastoid bone behind her right ear.

(　　) 4. There is a lot of bleeding from Ms. Yang's nose.

(　　) 5. Ms. Yang feels blood flowing back into her mouth.

(　　) 6. Ms. Yang looks healthy.

(　　) 7. Ms. Yang is fifty years old.

(　　) 8. Ms. Yang's nose bleeding may cause the obstruction of her ears.

New Words & Expressions

扫码听
单词

obstructed [əb'strʌktɪd]	adj. 阻塞的,梗阻的
purulent ['pjʊərʊlənt]	adj. 流脓的,化脓的
fetid ['fetɪd]	adj. 臭的,恶臭的
mastoid ['mæstɒɪd]	adj. 乳头状的
atherosclerosis [ˌæθərəʊsklə'rəʊsɪs]	n. 动脉粥样硬化

Conversation 2

扫码听
对话 2

Directions: <u>*Mrs. Wang has a great pain in her eyes*</u>. *She comes to the clinic for help. Fill in the blanks according to the conversation.*

(A：Nurse　B：Mrs. Wang)

A：Do you remember whether you were involved in any particular 1. _____ at that time?

B：I haven't noticed that.

A：Can you describe the whole course?

B：It started with seeing colored haloes around the white lights. My eyes were red and started 2. _____. Then I got a pain in the right eye, and it grew worse. At last I had a dull headache and couldn't see clearly. I felt sick and I have vomited several 3. _____.

A：Have you had anything like this before?

B：Yes, I've had several episodes like this before. But they were not so serious.

A：Does anything bring on these attacks?

B：I'm not sure, when I 4. _____ my temper or I felt very 5. _____ and so on.

A：How often do you get them?

B：It's difficult to say.

Note

A: Do you get them at night or in the day?

B: At night 6. _____ .

A: Have any of your family or immediate 7. _____ ever had similar problems?

B: My mother went 8. _____ with glaucoma when she was in her sixties.

A: Oh, I see. Let me measure your intraocular pressure with a tonometer.

New Words & Expressions

halo [ˈheɪləʊ]	n.	光晕
episode [ˈepɪsəʊd]	n.	一段经历,插曲
temper [ˈtempə(r)]	n.	脾气
glaucoma [glɔːˈkəʊmə]	n.	青光眼,绿内障
intraocular [ˌɪntrəˈɒkjʊlə]	adj.	眼内的
tonometer [təʊˈnɒmɪtə(r)]	n.	血压计,张力计

扫码听
单词

Group Discussion & Role Playing

1. Discuss with your partner. Change the patient types or demands and redesign the conversation.
2. Display the conversation you've made.
3. After one group finishes the performance, others make comments.

Intensive Reading

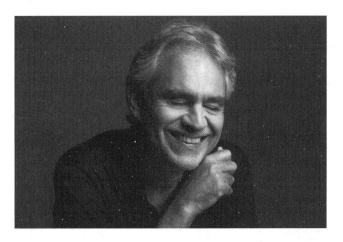

扫码听
课文

Turning Images into Sensations to Assist the Blind

Years ago, scientists began to learn that certain parts of the brain had certain duties. For example, one part was responsible for breathing; another dealt with the sense of smell. Scientists thought our brains could not change. But then they discovered that the brain could sometimes reorganize itself when conditions required. Josef Rauscheker is a professor of physiology and biophysics at Georgetown University in Washington. He wondered if this ability to change could

Note

explain the idea that other senses in blind people improve to balance their lack of vision. Professor Rauscheker and researchers from Finland and Belgium found this answer using an FMRI scanner. That means functional magnetic resonance imaging.

The machine recorded brain activity as twelve blind people and twelve sighted people performed tasks involving sound and touch. For example, they would try to decide which direction sounds were coming from, or which finger was feeling gentle vibrations. Professor Rauschecker says large parts of the visual cortex became active during the sound and touch texts, but only in the blind people. He says this study and earlier research have led to an experimental device designed to help the blind. It can process images taken by a camera into sensations that could be used by a blind person wearing it. Josef Rauschecker says, "So what we're hoping to do is build this device that would transform basically visual information into auditory information and then tap this amazing reservoir of the blind brain to process sounds and tactile information."

New Words & Expressions

扫码听
单词

reorganize [rɪˈɔːgənaɪz]	v. 整理,改组,重新制定
physiology [ˌfɪzɪˈɒlədʒɪ]	n. 生理学
biophysics [ˌbaɪəʊˈfɪzɪks]	n. 生物物理学
FMRI(Functional Magnetic Resonance Imaging)	功能性磁共振成像
scanner [ˈskænə(r)]	n. 扫描仪,扫描器
vibrations [ˈvaɪbreɪʃənz]	n. 振动,共鸣,动摇
visual cortex [ˈvɪʒuəl ˈkɔːteks]	n. 视皮质
auditory [ˈɔːdətrɪ]	adj. 听觉的
reservoir [ˈrezəvwɑː(r)]	n. 水库,蓄水池
tactile [ˈtæktaɪl]	adj. 触觉的,有触觉的,能触知的

Exercises

Exercise 1. Choose the best answer for each of the following questions.

1. Who is Josef Rauscheker? _____.

A. A scientist of medication

B. A doctor of ophthalmology and otorhinolaryngology

C. A professor of physiology and biophysics

D. A writer

2. How many people performed tasks involving sound and touch? _____.

A. 6   B. 24   C. 12   D. 30

3. What were the people asked to do in the sound and touch test? _____.

A. To record brain activity

B. To feel gentle vibration

C. To decide which finger was trembling

D. To decide which direction sounds were coming from

4. Whose visual cortex became active during the sound and touch texts? _____.

A. Musicians   B. Blind people   C. Average people   D. Sighted people

5. Which is not true about the experimental device? _____.

A. It can help the blind by wearing it

Note

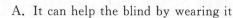

B. It can process images taken by a camera into sensations

C. It would transform auditory information into visual information

D. It would tap the amazing reservoir of the blind brain to process sounds and tactile information

Exercise 2. Decide whether the following statements are true (T) or false (F).

（　　）1. Different parts of the brain had certain duties.

（　　）2. The brain could not change itself when conditions required.

（　　）3. A large part of the visual cortex of the blind people became active during the sound and touch texts.

（　　）4. Scientists are hoping to build a device that would transform auditory information into visual information.

（　　）5. Researchers from Finland and Belgium found the answer by using an FMRI scanner.

Exercise 3. Fill in the blanks with the words given below, changing the form if necessary.

| visual | disproportionate | balance | gentle |
| designed | deal with | activity | stay |

1. But the increase in obesity（肥胖）has had a _____ impact on Americans' health and longevity（寿命）.

2. Children are supposed to get 60 minutes of physical _____ every day.

3. He was forced by his physical condition to _____ .

4. There are some _____ handicapped（残疾）boys and girls.

5. A psychiatrist（精神科医生）used hypnotism（催眠术）to help her _____ her fear.

Exercise 4. Arrange the following steps in a proper sequence based on the medical procedure.

1. Use a syringe device to gently direct water against the wall of the ear canal.

2. With the head upright，take hold of the outer part of the ear.

3. Then turn the head to the side to let the water out.

4. Gently pull upward to straighten the ear canal.

The correct order of ear care is：_____ .

Exercise 5. Translate the following Chinese sentences into English.

1. 今年春天一连串的自杀事件是由这次混乱引起的。

2. 尽量待在原地，我猜你的脚可能骨折了。

3. 放松一会儿就可以收获奇效。

4. 这次撞车事故涉及多少辆汽车？

5. 人适应环境的速度真是惊人。

Learning More

Ⅰ. Affixes & Roots of Medical Terms

Affixes & Roots	Chinese	More Words
cortic	皮层的	cortex 皮层；cortex corticis 肾皮质外层
cera	蜡	cerumen 耳垢；ceraceous 蜡状的

Note

Match the English expressions with the right Chinese phrases.

1. cerumen   A. 皮质类固醇

2. ceraceous   B. 肾皮质外层

3. corticosteroid   C. 蜡状的

4. cortex corticis   D. 耳垢

Ⅱ. Vocabulary Expansion

Match the Chinese phrases with the right English expressions.

A. cotton swab	B. irrigation	C. vibrations
D. resonance	E. sight	F. dizzy
G. symptom	H. mass	I. tap
J. irritant	K. ear canal	L. amplifier

1. (　　)共振   (　　)轻拍

2. (　　)耳道   (　　)视力

3. (　　)冲洗   (　　)使人头晕的

4. (　　)棉签   (　　)振动,共鸣

5. (　　)症状   (　　)块,团

Practical Writing

Resume(简历)

简历,也称履历,它是求职者向用人单位介绍其资格、职位、教育和工作经历等情况的文书,是求职和人才流动的重要文书,是求职者争取进一步面试的机会。其包括以下内容。

1. 个人资料:包括求职者的年龄、性别、身高、民族、出生地、婚姻状况、住址等。

2. 教育情况:一般只写大专(中专)以上的教育情况。中学的教育状况一般不要写上。

3. 工作经历:一般按照时间顺序写。

4. 重大成果或者著作、特长:列出成功的项目或出版的著作等。

Sample

Personal Resume

Basic information

Name：Li Yang   Gender：male

Date of birth：Jan. 4, 1999   Place of birth：Shanghai

Education and work experience

Educational background：Finished three-year study programme in Shanghai ×× College as an English major

Work experience：Conducted a three-month internship in ×× Primary School

Language ability：fluent Mandarin and English

续表

> **Job I am planning to apply for**：English teacher
>
> **Hobbies**：Reading and outdoor sports
>
> **Self-evaluation**：Have a strong sense of responsibility and team spirit
>
>
> Address：No. 21, Lane 12×× Road，×× District，Shanghai
>
> Post code：200210
>
> Phone：132××××××××

Exercise

Please write a resume according to the information given below.

【计划投简历给上海××医院，职位为护士】

Extended Knowledge

Ⅰ. First Aid—Treating minor burns

Step 1 Cool the burn.

Hold the burned area under cool (not cold) running water or apply a cool, wet compress until the pain eases.

Step 2 Remove rings or other tight items from the burned area.

Try to do this quickly and gently, before the area swells.

Step 3 Don't break blisters.

Fluid-filled blisters protect against infection. If a blister breaks, clean the area with water (mild soap is optional). Apply an antibiotic ointment. But if a rash appears, stop using the ointment.

Step 4 Apply lotion.

Once a burn is completely cooled, apply a lotion, such as one that contains aloe vera or a moisturizer. This helps prevent drying and provides relief.

Step 5 Bandage the burn.

Cover the burn with a sterile gauze bandage (not fluffy cotton). Wrap it loosely to avoid putting pressure on burned skin. Bandaging keeps air off the area, reduces pain and protects blistered skin.

Ⅱ. Knowledge Links

Dry eyes

Dry eyes are a common condition that occurs when your tears aren't able to provide adequate lubrication for your eyes. Tears can be inadequate for many reasons. For example, dry eyes may occur if you don't produce enough tears or if you produce poor-quality tears. Dry eyes feel uncomfortable. If you have dry eyes, your eyes may sting or burn. You may experience dry eyes in certain situations, such as on an airplane, in an air-conditioned room, while riding a bike or after looking at a computer screen for a few hours. Treatments for dry eyes may make you more comfortable. These treatments can include lifestyle changes and eyedrops. You'll likely need to take these measures indefinitely to control the symptoms of dry eyes.

扫码看
答案

Note

Scripts to Focus Listening

Unit 1

Conversation 1

Situation: Mr. Smith has been sleepless recently. He wants to see a doctor. But he finds that he cannot register online. So he makes a call for help.

(A: Nurse   B: Mr. Smith)

A: Hello, this is Patient Registration Department of People's Hospital.

B: Hello. I wonder if I could register for tomorrow morning. I cannot do it online.

A: I'm sorry, our system has just failed this morning. You cannot do it by yourself until tomorrow. Have you ever been here before?

B: No, this is my first visit.

A: Then tell me your basic information, please. I'll make an appointment for you.

B: That'll be nice. I'm John Smith, 38 years old. My insurance card number is 2770168.

A: OK. Which department do you want to register with?

B: I don't know exactly. I feel sleepless at night. It's difficult for me to fall asleep.

A: I think you should go to the Neurology Department first.

B: Fine. What time should I arrive there?

A: You'd better arrive here before 9:00 a. m. Please bring your ID card and insurance card.

B: OK. I'll go there on time. Thank you for your help.

A: You're welcome.

Conversation 2

Situation: Mr. Lin is calling to make an appointment at a doctor's office.

(A: Nurse   B: Mr. Lin)

A: Hello, this is Dr. Johnson's office. What can I do for you?

B: Hello. Can I make an appointment?

A: Sure. Have you been to see Dr. Johnson before?

B: Yes, I have. I had a physical checkup last year.

A: Fine. May I have your name?

B: Lin Fang.

A: OK, Mr. Lin. I've located your information. What's troubling you now?

B: I have some red spots on my arm, and it feels itchy. I think I need to have a check.

A: Do you need urgent care?

B: No, not necessarily, but I'd like to see the doctor soon.

A: Of course. The available time with Dr. Johnson will be 3:00 p. m. on Monday, 10:00 a. m. on

Tuesday, 8:00 a.m. on Wednesday. What is your convenient time?

B: I think 10:00 a.m. on Tuesday will be fine.

A: All right. Let me make your appointment at 10:00 a.m. on Tuesday with Dr. Johnson.

B: Thank you so much.

A: You are welcome. Bye.

B: Bye.

Unit 2

Conversation 1

Situation: A patient feels sick to his stomach. He is visiting a doctor in the consulting room.

(A: Doctor   B: Patient)

A: Good morning. What's troubling you?

B: It's my stomach. I think probably I had eaten too much at supper yesterday evening.

A: Can you tell me what you had for supper yesterday evening?

B: Seafood, roast duck. Oh, a great variety of things, I can't name them exactly.

A: Have you vomited?

B: Yes, I have vomited three times and made several trips to the bathroom last night.

A: I see. Now you have to get your stools tested. I'll write out a slip and you can take it to the laboratory. Wait for a while and pick up the report, and then bring it back to me.

B: All right, doctor. I'll see you later.

A: See you later.

B: Here's my report, Doctor.

A: Take your seat, and let me have a look. It's nothing serious, only indigestion due to too much oily food. I will prescribe you some medicine for it to make you feel better. I do advise you to avoid oily food for the next few days.

B: I will follow your advice. Thanks a lot.

A: You are welcome.

Conversation 2

Situation: A patient is visiting a doctor in the consulting room due to his cold.

(A: Doctor   B: Patient)

A: Good morning. What's troubling you?

B: Good morning , doctor. I think I have a cold.

A: How long have you been sick?

B: For two days.

A: What symptoms do you have?

B: I have a runny nose and I ache all over.

A: Do you have a fever?

B: I haven't taken my temperature yet, but I feel feverish.

A: Do you have a cough?

B: No, I don't.

A: Do you have a sore throat?

B: Yes, my throat feels swollen. It's sore.

A: I want to look at your throat. Open your mouth, please say "ah". It's only a common cold, nothing to worry about. You should rest for a few days and drink more water. I'll write you a certificate for three days' leave. Here is some Chinese traditional medicine, which is very effective for treating colds. You'll be fine in a few days.

B: Thanks a lot. Bye-bye!

A: Bye!

Unit 3

Conversation 1

Situation: Ms. Zheng has a prescription given by the doctor. She comes to the pharmacy for help.

(A: Chemist　B: Ms. Zheng)

A: Good morning. What can I do for you?

B: Good morning. Would you please fill the prescription for me?

A: Sure. Please wait for a moment.

B: OK.

A: Here is your herbal medicine.

B: Could you tell me how do I take the herbal medicine?

A: It's not difficult. First, place the herbs in a pot. Before decoction, soak the herbs in cold water for about twenty minutes, and then heat it up quickly. When it begins to boil, turn down the heat and simmer for thirty minutes. Then turn off the heat. Leave it to cool, and then pour out the liquid to drink. Be careful not to let any of the leaves go into the cup.

B: It seems a little complicated. Can I use a steel pan?

A: No, you can't do that. You'd better use an earthenware pot in order to prevent chemical changes.

B: Oh, I see.

A: Don't throw the herbs away. Do the same in the evening. That is the second dose. Take the first dose in the morning, the second in the evening.

B: Thank you very much.

A: You're welcome. I hope you will recover soon.

Conversation 2

Situation: Chen Hong has a bad cold. She comes to the pharmacy for help.

(A: Chemist　B: Chen Hong)

A: Good morning. May I help you?

B: Good morning. I have a terrible cold. Could you sell me some antibiotic medicine?

A: Do you have a prescription?

B: No, I haven't gone to see a doctor.

A: Sorry. I cannot sell it to you. You must first get a doctor's prescription, and then I can fill it for you. But I can recommend some OTC medicine to relieve the symptoms of cold.

B: I see. Could you suggest something I can take to relieve the headache?

A: We have a number of painkillers. They are all very good. How about this brand?

B: All right. How do I take this medicine?

A: Take one tablet whenever you feel pain, but do not take more than three times a day.

B: Thank you very much.

A: You're welcome. I hope you will recover soon.

Unit 4

Conversation 1

Situation: Mr. Smith is going to be admitted to the hospital. Now he is talking with the nurse about something important for admission.

(A: Nurse   B: Mr. Smith)

A: Good morning. What can I do for you?

B: Good morning. I'm here for admission to the hospital.

A: Would you please show me your admission form, please?

B: Here you are.

A: OK. Let's get started now. After filling in this form, I will bring you to the ward.

B: Well, wait a minute, please.

A: OK. And now we are taking the elevator, and then walk over to the yellow wing of the hospital which you can see over there. Let me help you to carry this bag.

B: All right. I didn't intend to bring many things just for three days stay. But then again it all mounts up and I have hand to bring two suitcases after all.

A: Don't worry. We can offer those things that you need, such as slippers and toothbrush. What's more, there are some shops on the fourth floor.

B: It sounds good. I will go around if I need it.

Conversation 2

Situation: Mrs. Wang is in the ward. Now the nurse is introducing the surrounding of the ward to her.

(A: Nurse   B: Mrs. Wang)

A: Hello, Mrs. Wang.

B: Hello, nice meeting you.

A: This is the tub and shower room. You can use it from 7 o'clock in the morning to 8 o'clock in the evening. Here is a toilet. Another one is over there, in case this one is occupied. This bed is yours, and this is your call button. If you need any help, you can push the button once, like this. When you call us, a light will be on outside your room, and we will come into the ward to help you. Do you understand my explanation?

B: Yes, I do. Thank you.

A: This is your bedside table. You'd better keep only small things that you need often, such as toilet articles and some underwear. The valuables can put in the hospital safe if you wish. Any questions?

B: No, I don't. Many thanks.

A: Would you mind changing into your nightgown? Your doctor will come to see you later. I'll be back in a few minutes.

Unit 5

Conversation 1

Situation: Doctor Murray is doing a physical test for Mark.

（A：Doctor Murray B：Mark）

A：OK, Mark. We need to do a couple of tests. The first one is your thyroid function test.

B：What's that? I think you told me last time but I've forgotten. There was so much to understand.

A：It tests how well your thyroid is working. We think it's working a bit too well and we want to check. Clear? Any questions?

B：I'm sorry. What's my thyroid?

A：OK, Let's start from the beginning. Your thyroid gland, in some ways, is like the accelerator on a car. It controls how fast your system works and lots of other things as well. The thyroid gland produces a hormone, that's a chemical messenger, called thyroxin. If there is too much in your blood, your system goes too quickly, if there is not enough it goes too slowly. Do you follow?

B：Sure.

A：So if the thyroid gland is like the accelerator, thyroxin is like the gas.

B：But what has this got to do with my diabetes?

A：Well, you remember last time I told you that carbohydrate makes your blood sugar go up, while insulin and exercise keep your blood sugar levels down...

B：Sure, that's why I have to reduce my insulin if I do a lot of exercise. But it is really difficult to balance them.

A：Well, this is where the thyroid comes in. It's really difficult to keep your blood sugar right if your thyroid gland keeps putting its foot on the accelerator.

B：And I'm trying to put my foot on the brake at the same time.

A：OK! So you see why we have to keep checking your thyroid function.

B：Yes, that's much clearer.

A：OK! Mark, I'm sure you understood but just to check, can you run through it again for me?

B：OK.

Conversation 2

Situation: Robert is calling the hospital in California where Mrs. Marshall received treatment ten days ago.

（A：Dr. Kim B：Robert）

A：Hello, may I help you?

B：Hi, is that Dr. Kim?

A：Speaking.

B：Good Morning, Dr. Kim. This is Robert Mitchell speaking from Ashville Hospital. We have a patient here whom you treated about 10 days ago. She has presented with a stroke and we would like to check up on the treatment she had with you.

A：Sure. What's the patient's name?

B：Mrs. Linda Marshall, aged 62.

A：OK, let me check the computer. OK, here we are. Retired factory worker, a patient with myocardial infarction. Right?

B: Right.

A: OK, she presented with chest pain. The electrocardiogram showed ST segment and T wave abnormality but there was no Q wave abnormality.

B: OK, let me just write that down. Chest pain. No Q wave abnormality but ST segment and T wave abnormality. Diagnosis: myocardial infarction. OK.

A: Right. We gave her the usual acute MI medications: I. V. morphine, aspirin and heparin and put her under observation.

B: OK, so we have intra-venous morphine, aspirin and heparin. OK.

A: She responded very well and after six hours her T waves were looking much better.

B: That's good. Thank you Dr. Kim. Good to talk to you.

A: You're welcome, Robert. Hope the case goes well.

Unit 6

Conversation 1

Situation: Bed 22, is Wang Hua, 50 years old, under Dr. Li. She was admitted late yesterday afternoon with a lump in her right breast. She's going to have a fine-needle biopsy this afternoon. Now she is talking to Miss Chen, her nurse in charge on the ward.

(A: Wang Hua B: Miss Chen)

A: Excuse me, Miss Chen, can I have a word with you?

B: Sure.

A: I'm having a test this afternoon and I don't know what exactly it is. I'm worried about it. Could you explain it to me?

B: I'm sure you are clear about your problem.

A: I've got a lump in my right breast.

B: OK. Well, you are having a fine-needle biopsy.

A: Could you tell me more about the test?

B: They use a syringe and they pull back on it and get some of the fluid and some of the cells. After that they send it off to a pathology and cytology lab to check on the cells.

A: When can I get the results?

B: You probably won't find out until tomorrow or later than that.

A: I am wondering whether I need an operation if the results turn out to be negative?

B: Well, if the results come back as all clear, then you won't need an operation.

A: OK and if it's not all clear?

B: Well, your doctor has prescribed you ultrasound test which is to be done tomorrow. So we shall wait for the results of both those tests. The doctor will decide whether you need an operation or not according to the results.

A: So basically we shall wait and see.

B: Yeah, unfortunately, it is, yes.

A: I got it. Thanks for your explanation.

Conversation 2

Situation: Ms. Wang is a 43-year-old woman who is now in her 31st week of pregnancy. She has been hospitalized recently for occasional headache. She was diagnosed as hypertensive disorders in pregnancy. Now she complains that her headache is much more serious when the nurse Miss Li comes into the ward.

(A: Ms. Wang　B: Miss Li, the nurse)

A: Miss Li, do you mind coming here and having a look at me?

B: Ms. Wang, what is happening?

A: My headache is much more serious now, and I can't endure this any longer.

B: Let me help you to lie down, then I'll take your blood pressure and heart rate.

A: OK, thank you.

B: Your blood pressure is 160/110 which is higher than normal and heart rate is 90 beats/min. I'll check your legs to see if you have edema. Please bend your legs. (*Nurse presses both legs.*)

A: How about my legs?

B: Yes, edema really exists on both legs.

A: How about my urine test and blood test in the morning? Have the results come out?

B: Yes, both the results have come out. Here you are. The urine report tells that urinary protein is beyond the normal range and the blood reports shows that you are anemic.

A: Is that very serious?

B: More foods rich in iron are suggested. By the way, I've checked the doctor's order. There is still several hours to go for your next dose. I'll notify the doctor your situation.

A: Thank you, Miss Li.

B: You are welcome.

Unit 7

Conversation 1

Situation: The patient Roy has been in trouble of weight problem. She comes to the doctor for help.

(A: Doctor　B: Patient)

A: According to your test result... well... Roy, your BMI is 32.8, and that means you really should take care of your weight problem.

B: You're saying I'm overweight?

A: More than that, you know, BMI equals a person's weight in kilograms divided by height in meters squared. For adults 35 and older, having a BMI greater than 30 is considered obese.

B: Oh, no, doctor! This could not be happening to me. I have been exercising for weeks and tried many ways to cut down weight... just don't work!

A: Don't worry. There are many reasons for obesity, for example, genetics. A person is more likely to develop obesity if one or both parents are obese. Genetics also affect hormones involved in fat regulation. And other factors may be overeating, slow metabolism and so on.

B: Yeah, right, doctor. My father used to have the same thing and also many other related problems.

A: Obesity does lead to many health problems, such as insulin resistance, type 2 diabetes, hypertension, stroke, heart attack and sleep apnea, etc. So...

B: These days my blood pressure is not steady and sometimes it is abnormally high. And is there any way to tackle my problem?

A: Here is the treatment package I offer you: Perform 20-30 minutes of moderate exercise five to seven days a week, including walking, stationary bicycling, walking or jogging on a treadmill, stair climbing machines, jogging, and swimming. For you, I will also recommend some other medicines.

B: Thank you.

Conversation 2

Situation: Mrs. King has been retired for several years and she starts to lose her memory. She comes to the doctor for help.

(A: Doctor   B: Patient)

A: Hello, Mrs. King. How are you today?

B: Oh, I'm fine, very well, thank you.

A: You know who I am, don't you?

B: Now, let me see now. I know your face, but I can't quite place who you are. I think I know. I think I should know who you are.

A: Well, I'm Dr. Williams. I've met you many times before, you know.

B: Oh, you're the doctor. Well I remember old Dr. Wang quite well, but I don't remember seeing him recently.

A: No, Dr. Wang has been retired for several years. I took over his practice and I've seen you before. Maybe you don't recall that. Have you been here long?

B: Where, where do you mean?

A: In this house, have you been here long?

B: Oh, I've been here sometime I think.

A: Do you remember where this is? Where is this place?

B: This is the High Street, isn't it?

A: Yes, this is the High Street. How long have you been living in the High Street?

B: Oh, it must be a good number of years now. My father used to stay down in North High Street of course, and I used to stay with him, but when I got married, I moved up here. Oh, that must be a good number of years, I can't quite remember the time.

A: Do you remember when you were born? What was the year of your birth? Can you remember that?

B: Oh, yes. I was born in 1941.

A: Well, very good, Mrs. King, how old will you be now, do you think?

B: Oh, I've retired now. I must be about 67. Sorry, I'm not sure.

A: Well, there's no doubt the years go by.

Unit 8

Conversation 1

Situation: In the Out-patient Department, Andrew is brought to the hospital for a sports accident.

(A: Doctor   B: Andrew)

A: What's wrong with you, Andrew?

B: My foot is hurt when I was playing basketball. I'm in so much pain now.

A: Oh, let me have a look at the hurt foot. Does it hurt when I do this?

B: Ouch! It hurts so much! I bet I am going to lose my foot!

A: Don't worry, Andrew. I'll check your foot. Now lie on the bed. Your injured foot looks a little blue. Can you move it?

B: Yes, a little.

A: Can you describe your pain? Is it there all the time or it only hurts when you move it?

B: It's there all the time.

A: I see. Now could you give me a number to rate your pain? 1 is no pain and 10 is the worst pain imaginable. What number would you give me?

B: 8 at least.

A: That must be really hurting. Now I'm going to check your pulses. The pulse of the injured one is a little faster. But don't worry, there is no fracture. What you need is a wrap and crutches for ambulation.

Conversation 2

Situation: Getting the doctor's advice in Conversation 1, the nurse is giving Andrew a wrap and instructing him to use crutches.

(A: Nurse   B: Andrew)

A: Now let me help you with a wrap. Finished! Let me check your pulse again. Oh, it is better, and the color is better, too.

B: Yes, I feel much better too.

A: OK, to help you get enough support, I'll teach you how to use crutches. Can you sit up by yourself? Well done! Do you feel dizzy now?

B: No.

A: OK, now I'll help you put on your shoes. Are they tight?

B: No.

A: Good. Now please hold the crutches and I'll help you adjust them to your proper height. On a count of three, I'll help you stand up. One, two, three. OK, how do you feel now?

B: Well, comfortable.

A: Good. To use the crutches properly, you must make sure to put your weight on the handles but not on your arms. Would you please have a try?

B: Like this?

A: Yes. When you are standing with crutches, all weight is on the good leg. That's right. When you are walking, you should move both crutches first, and then the strong foot. That's right. Do you have any questions?

B: I don't think so.

A: OK, please use the crutches to walk at home.

B: OK, thank you, nurse. Goodbye.

A: See you.

Unit 9

Conversation 1

Situation: A nurse is examining Linda, a first-time mother, who is having labor pains.

(A: Nurse   B: Linda)

A: Good morning, Linda!

B: Good morning.

A: How are you feeling this morning?

B: I'm starting to have labor pains.

A: Oh, take it easy. How often do the pains come and how long do they last?

B: About every 20 minutes and they last for 10 seconds.

A: OK. Every contraction means the baby is coming one step nearer to you. Relaxation helps to relieve the pain. You can do something interesting to distract yourself from the pain. Let's say, imagine what your baby looks like.

B: The baby must look like me.

A: We'll know the answer soon. Now I will check your hourly pulse, blood pressure and temperature. Please choose a position you are comfortable with.

B: I'm not comfortable lying down. My back aches.

A: Let me place a pillow under your hips. Feel better now?

B: Yes, much better.

A: You can ask your family to massage your back to relieve the pain.

B: OK. When am I to give birth?

A: You are not in strong labor yet. You'd better try to get on with everyday life. You can eat, drink, walk or even watch a film. Just relax! Linda.

B: How long does it take to get into the next stage?

A: This varies from person to person. It's hard to say. As the labor advances, the contractions become stronger and increasingly painful. You may close your eyes and breathe deeply and rhythmically, or even moan or call out when you feel you can't endure the pain. But I'm always at your call to help you.

B: This is my first baby. I'm really nervous.

A: To be a mother is to be strong. Your baby is just on the way, Linda. From now on, time your contractions carefully. When they come every 10 minutes and last 20 to 30 seconds, tell us, please.

Conversation 2

Situation: A doctor is in the pediatric consulting room. She is having a conversation with the patient, Tom and his mother.

(A: Doctor   B: Tom's mother   C: Tom)

A: Good afternoon. How can I help you?

B: My child has a temperature, headache, sore throat and rash.

A: How long has he been ill?

B: He's had the temperature since yesterday.

A: (Turns to the child) Tom, let me have a look. Open your mouth and show me your tongue.

C: No. I have a sore throat.

A: Tom, I know how you are feeling now. See those cute stickers? They are for brave kids.

C: Emmm... OK. Ah...

B: What have you found?

A: His tonsils are swollen and red. His tongue is as red as a strawberry. There is a rash all over his body. A blood test is necessary.

(*After a while*)

A: Here comes the result.

B: Is it normal, doctor?

A: His white blood cell count is high. He is probably having a scarlet fever.

B: Scarlet fever? What kind of disease is it?

A: It is a kind of infectious disease. You should keep him away from other children as soon as possible.

B: What can I do to help him recover soon?

A: He should stay in bed until his fever goes down. Easily digestible food is preferred and drinking plenty of fluids is a must.

B: What drugs does he have to take?

A: Penicillin injections for a few days.

B: What should I do to protect his sister?

A: She'd better stay far away from Tom and wear a mask if possible.

B: I got it. Thank you.

Unit 10

Conversation 1

Situation: Ms. Li has been sneezing, nose stuffing and itching recently. She comes to the TCM for help.

(A: Doctor   B: Ms. Li)

A: Hello, Ms. Li. What can I do for you?

B: I've been sneezing, nose stuffing and itching.

A: Do you have a fever or cough?

B: No. I thought it was a cold at the beginning, so I took cold medicine for a week, but it didn't work. Therefore, I'm here now.

A: Then do you feel itchy in the eyes?

B: Yes, not only the eyes, but also I feel uncomfortable in the mouth.

A: You have allergic rhinitis. First of all, it is recommended that you go to allergy department to find out your allergens, stay away from the allergens and take some desensitization drugs. You can relieve the allergic symptoms by this way. But if you want to cure the allergy, you should choose immunotherapy. In this TCM department, I recommend you to receive dog day moxibustion treatment every year.

B: What is dog day moxibustion treatment?

A: dog day moxibustion treatment is based on the TCM theory of "treating winter diseases in summer". It is to apply herbal products to specific acupoints in the hottest dog days to stimulate Yang Qi, dispel inner cold and treat winter diseases. The properties of the herbs are warm, suitable for slowly conditioning body and enhancing immunity.

B: What diseases can it cure?

A: Respiratory diseases, such as asthma and bronchitis; ENT diseases, such as allergic rhinitis, rheumatic diseases and so on.

B: Is it suitable for children?

A: Sure.

B: That's great. I can bring my child here. When should I have the plasters?

A: On the first day of the dog days. Three times in total each year.

B: OK. I'll be sure to come then. Thank you, doctor.

Conversation 2

Situation: Ms. Wang has been losing her sleep and appetite. She comes to the TCM department for help.

(A: Doctor   B: Ms. Wang)

A: Hello, please have a seat.

B: I've been losing my sleep and my appetite.

A: How long have you been like this?

B: About two months. It really tortures me a lot.

A: Are there any other discomforts?

B: Headache, and sometimes dizziness.

A: Have you taken any medicine?

B: Yes. I've been taking western medicines these days, but I am also worried about their side effects, so I want to try Chinese herbal medicine.

A: All right. Please give me your hand and I'll take your pulse.

(*During pulse diagnosis...*)

A: You have wiry and rapid pulse. Are you in a bad mood recently? Do you always get angry?

B: Yes.

A: Do you have bitter taste in your mouth?

B: Yes.

A: Let me have a look at your tongue, please.

(*Pulse examination is completed.*)

A: You have red tongue with yellow coating. According to your symptoms, this is caused by stagnated liver-Qi changing into fire. You need to disperse stagnated liver-Qi, eliminate heat, and calm the mind. I'll give you some Chinese herbs for internal use. In addition, you also need acupuncture. Internal and external conditioning can recover your body gradually.

B: All right.

A: This is your prescription. Please get the herbs at the pharmacy. They can help you to decoct the herbs into patent medicine if you like. This is your acupuncture schedule.

B: Thank you very much.

A: You're welcome.

Unit 11

Conversation 1

Situation: Mrs. Smith has been hospitalized six days after the operation and she needs to get nutrition by tube feeding. A nurse comes to inform her of the performance of tube feeding.

(A: Nurse   B: Mrs. Smith)

A: Hello! Mrs. Smith. How are you today?

B: Not too bad, thanks.

A: That looks like an interesting program you're watching.

B: Yes, I like it. That helps me kill time.

A: Mrs. Smith, I'm afraid I have to put a tube through your nose to your stomach now.

B: It sounds awful!

A: I know. It's not very pleasant, but I'll try to make you as comfortable as possible. Besides, according to the doctor's order, it is necessary for you to get enough nutrition by tube feeding 6 days after the operation.

B: All right.

A: I'll show you everything that I'm going to use, so you'll understand what's happening.

B: OK.

A: I'll just turn off the TV so we're not distracted. Then I'll draw the curtain to keep your privacy.

B: OK. Thanks.

A: Here's the tube which goes into your stomach.

B: Ooh, it's very long.

A: That's because it has to go in through your nose and down into your stomach.

B: I see, but I feel it extremely unbearable to let it go into my belly.

A: Don't worry. I will feed the tube through your nose softly and carefully. All you need to do is to swallow it as I tell you.

B: I'm really nervous about this. I don't know if I can do it. It seems impossible.

A: It's OK. During the process, you tend to feel uneasy. Mark my words. I'll stop if you need a break. Just hold up your hand and I'll stop right away.

B: You will?

A: Yes. Just hold up your hand and I'll stop. Just as I said, I'll try to make you as comfortable as I can.

B: Right. I feel a bit better about it now.

A: All right. If I start now?

B: Yes, go ahead.

Conversation 2

Situation: Mr. Silverman can't manage to take a bath alone because of the fraction. A nurse comes to instruct him how to do it by himself.

(A: Nurse   B: Mr. Silverman)

A: Hello, Mr. Silverman. Did you have a good sleep last night?

B: Awful. I had a shocking night. I didn't sleep a wink.

A: That's no good. Do you know why? Were you in pain?

B: No, no pain at all. But I smelt so stinky. I went to sleep without taking a bath.

A: Oh, really? What was happening?

B: I was useless. I was unable to go into the bathtub and take a bath by myself.

A: Don't worry. I am going to teach you how to transfer from the wheelchair to the bathtub by yourself.

B: Oh, OK. That would be amazing if possible.

A: You need a transfer board and a stool if you want to manage it yourself. Here are the transfer board and the stool, which is as high as the tub.

B: Sorry, what are they for?

A: Let's take them to the bathroom. I'd like to show you how to use them.

B: All right.

A: Here we are. First, have your wheelchair stand against the tub side by side.

B: Is that right?

A: Yes. Then put the stool into the tub.

B: OK. And then?

A: Here comes the next step. Put one end of the transfer board on your wheelchair and the other on the stool. The transfer board functions as a sliding board.

B: Is that OK?

A: Mm. OK. You have to make sure the transfer board is rather balanced.

B: All right. What goes next?

A: The next step is to lift your legs with your hands and put them into the tub one by one.

B: OK. That is done.

A: You have to take it easy. Don't rush. Otherwise, your legs tend to get hurt.

B: I'll do that. Then what should I do?

A: It is vital. You slide with your bottom from the wheelchair onto the transfer board and then move along the transfer board onto the stool. Yes, that's right.

B: Wow, I made it. I am in the tub. Thank you so much.

A: You're welcome. You did a wonderful job. Finally, I'd like you to remember to take it slowly next time you do it.

B: I'll do exactly as you tell me to. Thanks again.

A: That's nothing. Enjoy your bath. Goodbye.

B: Bye.

Unit 12

Conversation 1

Situation: Ms. Yang has got a pain and a purulent flow in her ear. She comes to the otolaryngology department for help.

(A: Nurse   B: Ms. Yang)

A: What's wrong with you?

B: My right ear seems to be obstructed.

A: Is your hearing affected? Do you have ringing in the ear?

B: Yes, in the right ear.

A: Have you got any pain in your ear?

B: Yes, I have got an earache.

A: Do you have an ear flow?

B: Yes, there is a purulent flow.

A: What is the odor of this flow?

B: It is rather fetid.

A: Do you feel pain when I press on the mastoid bone behind your right ear?

B: A little.

A: Do you have any sense of dizziness?

B: Yes, very often.

A: Since when have you been feeling like this?

B: It all started the day before yesterday.

A：Well，let me examine your ear.

(*After the examination...*)

A：Oh，there is also massive bleeding from your nose.

B：Yes，my nose often bleeds.

A：Let me insert cotton balls in your nose to stop bleeding.

B：Now I feel better. Thank you.

A：Do you have any blood in your mouth?

B：Yes，I feel blood flowing back into my mouth and my ears.

A：You look quite unhealthy. How old are you?

B：I'm sixty.

A：How about your blood pressure?

B：160/110 mmHg. I also have atherosclerosis.

A：Let me examine your nose and throat. Bleeding in your nose may be the main cause of the obstruction of your ears.

Conversation 2

Situation：Ms. Wang has a great pain in her eyes. She comes to the clinic for help.

(A：Nurse   B：Ms. Wang)

A：What's your trouble?

B：My eyes are feeling a great pain and I can't stand it anymore. Please kill the pain for me right away!

A：Are both eyes affected?

B：Only the right one.

A：How long has it lasted?

B：For two hours.

A：Do you remember whether you were involved in any particular activity at that time?

B：I haven't noticed that.

A：Can you describe the whole course?

B：It started with seeing colored haloes around the white lights. My eyes were red and started running. Then I got a pain in the right eye，and it grew worse. At last I had a dull headache and couldn't see clearly. I felt sick and I have vomited several times.

A：Have you had anything like this before?

B：Yes,I've had several episodes like this before. But they were not so serious.

A：Does anything bring on these attacks?

B：I'm not sure，when I lost my temper or I felt very tired and so on.

A：How often do you get them?

B：It's difficult to say.

A：Do you get them at night or in the day?

B：At night usually.

A：Have any of your family or immediate relatives ever had similar problems?

B：My mother went blind with glaucoma when she was in her sixties.

A：Oh，I see. Let me measure your intraocular pressure with a tonometer.

Translations of Intensive Reading

Unit 1

人体系统

从生物学上来说,人体是由多个系统构成的,这些身体系统在我们每天的生活中发挥着各自的作用。了解这些系统有助于我们了解身体系统是如何运作的,理解为什么保持健康对我们的生活这么重要。

皮肤系统

皮肤系统是保护我们免受细菌和病毒侵害的屏障。它还能调节体温,通过汗液代谢废物。除了皮肤之外,皮肤系统还包括头发和指甲。

呼吸系统

呼吸系统参与的是呼吸过程。肺作为呼吸过程中的主要器官,负责吸入氧气,呼出二氧化碳,实现气体交换。

循环系统

循环系统是由心脏、血液和血管组成的网络结构。这个网络为细胞提供营养和氧气,并清除废物。我们的饮食和运动习惯可能会影响我们的循环系统。

肌肉骨骼系统

肌肉骨骼系统,与人体的肌肉和骨骼相关。它为身体提供支撑、稳定和运动的功能。

消化系统

消化系统由分解食物、吸收营养和排泄废物的器官组成。大多数消化器官形成了一个长而连续的消化道。还有一些消化道外的附属器官如肝、胰腺。

内分泌系统

内分泌系统的重要功能是分泌和调节激素。大多数内分泌疾病是由于激素过多或过少引起的,包括糖尿病、甲状腺功能亢进和甲状腺功能减退。

神经系统

神经系统是一个复杂的网络,它向身体的各个部位传递信号。从结构上看,它由中枢神经系统(CNS)和周围神经系统(PNS)组成。

生殖系统

生殖系统的主要功能是繁殖和产生后代。该系统的激素分泌异常等问题经常影响生育能力。

泌尿系统

泌尿系统清除血液中的有害废物并以尿液的形式排出体外。通过这样的方式来保持我们的身体健康。肾脏过滤出来的废液被储存在膀胱里,然后将其排出体外。

Unit 2

门　诊　部

门诊患者

门诊患者是到医院或诊所看病而不需要在就诊处过夜的人。通常情况下门诊的就诊过程简单而快捷,患者可以自己进出医院或者诊所。很多人在他们生命中的某个阶段都曾接受过门诊治疗,每一次你去医生诊室做检查、看感冒或祛痣时,你就是门诊患者。

门诊手术

门诊手术是指那些通常不需要患者在完成手术后在医院过夜的手术。大多数人做完简单的门诊手术后几个小时就回家了。事实上,门诊手术的数量呈增加的趋势。门诊手术为什么更受欢迎且更安全有如下几个原因。

首先,手术技术在过去几十年里越来越成熟。有些手术甚至不需要很大的切口,这意味着手术创伤的风险极小。麻醉技术也在不断改善,使人们更容易地从全身麻醉中快速恢复过来,而且没有并发症。研究还表明,许多人在家里比在医院康复得更好,在医院可能会比较吵闹而且易增加感染的风险。门诊手术增加的另一个驱动力是它降低了医疗成本。住院治疗既昂贵又复杂。当住院不是必须的时候,成本就会明显减少。

门诊药房

门诊药房是为其所属医疗机构患者配药的药房,通常是医院或诊所。为了方便患者,医院通常提供门诊药房服务。

与普通药房相比,对患者来说门诊药房有几个优势:第一,门诊药房就在他们接受治疗的地方,所以他们不需要额外跑一趟药房取药;第二,门诊药房的工作人员通常对患者的情况非常了解,他们能够迅速发现潜在的药物冲突和其他可能出现的问题;第三,门诊药房也可以提供优惠的价格。

Unit 3

怎样正确给药

药物在预防、诊断和治疗疾病中起着重要作用。为了促进患者的健康,医护人员必须采用正确的给药方法和途径才能达到应有的治疗效果。

1. 给药前,请先核对"五准确"。

首先,你要核对"五准确"。"五准确"指准确的患者,准确的药,准确的剂量,准确的给药途径和准确的时间及频次。例如,在询问患者姓名的同时,询问他的出生日期,以确保处方与患者匹配。

2. 在给服任何新药之前,请询问患者对药物的过敏史和反应情况。

3. 避免缩写,在记录药物过敏时缩写很容易被误解。

4. 密切注意患者的关键诊断,以及患者的吸烟、饮酒和药品使用情况等,这些不仅会影响药物的选择,还会影响剂量和服用频次,尤其是患有肾脏、肝脏、精神疾病和糖尿病的患者以及孕妇。

5. 注意患者目前的用药方案,并在每次就诊时更新清单。这应该被记录在他的表上的相同位置,以便于查找。你不仅应记录处方药,还应记录任何非处方药、中草药或补品的剂量和服用频次。

6. 学习并区分相似的药物名称。大多数药物名称听起来很相似但用途不同。例如,药物 Celebrex(西乐葆)通常用于治疗关节炎,而相似名称的 Cerebyx(磷苯妥英)用于治疗癫痫发作。

7. 将需要"高度警惕"或听起来相似的药品存放在不同的区域,以免混淆。确保药物存放区井井有条,至少每季度检查一次药物存储区域,丢弃所有过期的药物,并确保药物标签易于阅读并面向货架。

Unit 4

入　院

为了评估患者临床状况和护理需要,患者不可避免地要办理入院手续,这也是收集资料的一种方法。

入院前的准备和登记

患者来办理入院手续时,请检查以下项目。

1. 主治医生会为患者提供入院卡/入院通知。因为只有凭医生的建议,患者才可入院治疗。

2. 提供包含个人资料、病史、入院原因和将采取的治疗等内容的入院表格也是必要的。

3. 患者最好带上身份证、国家健康保险 IC 卡及相关的证明。

4. 患者必须带上以前的医疗记录、化验结果、X 线检查结果以及目前正在服用的药物清单。

5. 患者需提前交付押金。

入院程序

1. 当挂号处确定了患者何时可以入院后,护士将电话通知患者具体的入院时间。患者或其家属应在通知的时间内办理好所有的住院手续,否则将不予保留床位。

2. 患者需要自己带内衣和日常生活用品。患者须谨记:住院期间请勿携带贵重物品。

3. 到达医院

入院当天请携带上述所有物品,并把它们交给住院处。患者需要在住院协议上签字,然后被领到各自的病房。

4. 到达病房

患者到达病房后,医务人员会向患者介绍病房的情况,并即刻为其提供医疗护理服务。患者到达后将会被护送到分配的病床,病房小组成员将帮助患者熟悉周围环境。

为了获得患者的简明医疗史和社交史,护士将会来问患者一系列问题。为了帮助麻醉师计算所需药物的剂量,护士会测量患者的体重和身高。此外,护士还将测量患者的血压、心率、血氧饱和度和体温。这是手术前的基准测量。

Unit 5

放　射　学

放射学是与 X 射线研究有关的医学专业。X 射线是由能量源(X 射线机或阴极射线管)产生的不可见能量波。X 射线的一些特征对医生的疾病诊断和治疗很有帮助。

它的一些特征:

1. 能够引起照相底片曝光。如果将底片放置在 X 射线束的前面,则 X 射线不受阻碍地在空气中传播,将使底片的银涂层暴露出来并使其变黑。

2. 能够不同程度地渗透不同物质。X 射线可以轻松通过人体中不同类型的物质。如果 X 射线被人体物质(如骨骼中的钙)吸收(阻止),则 X 射线不会到达患者身后的照相板,并且 X 射线胶片(板)中会留下白色区域。

3. 隐形性。X 射线不能被视觉、听觉或触觉探测到。接触 X 射线的工作人员必须佩戴一个胶片式射线计量器,它包含一种被 X 射线照射的特殊胶片,胶片中的黑度表示佩戴者所接收的 X 射线或伽马射线的数量。

X 射线以多种方式用于检测病理状况。其最常见的用途是在牙科检查中,用以定位牙齿中的蛀牙。其他的检查区域包括消化系统、神经系统、生殖系统、内分泌系统以及胸部和骨骼。

Unit 6

医 学 检 验

　　医学检验是指为检测、诊断或监测疾病、疾病过程、易感性和确定治疗过程而进行的一种医学程序。它与临床化学和分子诊断有关,通常在医学实验室进行。医学检验用途广泛。当接诊患者时,医生会开出单子让患者进行常规检查,以检查某些疾病,或监测他们的健康。在一些情况下,它们也是就业的必要条件。

　　一般来说,我们熟悉的常见医学检验包括血液检查、病理检查、血糖检查、基因检测、胆固醇检测和内镜检查。根据不同的标准,医学检验可以分为不同的类型。根据检测样本,医学检验分为血液检测、尿液检测、粪便检测和痰检。以上提及的常见检查包括在患者的排尿量增加一段时间后,对疑似糖尿病患者进行血糖检查;对高热患者进行全血计数,确认是否有细菌感染;监测胸痛患者的心电图读数,诊断任何心脏疾病。

　　诚然,一些医学检验程序确实会对健康造成一定的风险,甚至需要对受试者进行麻醉,但最常见的医学检验,如血液检测或妊娠检测,几乎没有或根本没有直接风险。

Unit 7

心碎综合征

　　心碎综合征,也被称为压力诱发的心肌病,即使你是健康的,也会发作。

　　与男性相比,女性更有可能经历由情绪压力事件引起的突发、剧烈的胸痛,这是应激激素激增的反应。它可以是爱人的死亡,或者是离婚、分手等。它甚至可能发生在一次良好的冲击之后。

　　心碎综合征可能被误诊为心脏病发作,因为症状和检测结果与心脏病相似。事实上,测试显示,心脏病发作的典型症状是心率和血液中的物质会发生剧烈变化。但与心脏病发作不同,在心碎综合征中没有心脏动脉阻塞的证据。

　　在心碎综合征中,你的心脏的一部分会暂时增大,泵血功能不佳,而你的心脏的其他部分则会正常运作,甚至出现更强烈的收缩。研究人员才刚刚开始了解其原因以及如何对其诊断和治疗。

　　坏消息是心碎综合征会导致严重的、短期的心肌衰竭。

　　好消息是心碎综合征通常是可以治疗的。大多数经历过的人在几周内就能完全康复,再次发生这种情况的风险也很低(虽然在极少数情况下可能是致命的)。

　　应该注意的是迹象和症状。

　　心碎综合征最常见的症状是心绞痛(胸痛)和气短。即使你没有心脏病史,你也可能经历这些事情。

　　心律失常或心源性休克也可能发生在心碎综合征中。心源性休克是一种突然变弱的心脏无法泵出足够的血液来满足身体需要的情况,如果不立即治疗,可能是致命的。当人们死于心脏病发作时,心源性休克是最常见的死亡原因。

Unit 8

如何应对观察等待期的焦虑情绪

　　如果你被诊断出患有癌症,你的肿瘤医生可能会建议你"观察等待"一段时间。观察等待对你而言可能是心理上的挑战,这取决于你的诊断和积极治疗(化疗、放疗或手术)的时间。

　　你可能担心在等待的过程中癌症会发展和扩散;你可能会感到焦虑,因为在你等待的过程中医生

"无所作为";或者你可能会觉得被困住了,看到观察等待结束时的扫描或检查结果你才能回归正常生活。倾听他人的经历可以帮助你形成适合自己的应对策略。贝丝的故事可能会给你一些有用的见解。

贝丝被诊断为左乳Ⅰ期乳腺癌,并接受了手术和放疗。在一次常规术后检查中,乳房 X 线片显示右乳房上有一个可能有问题的斑点。令她惊讶的是,她的肿瘤医生并没有建议她立即对右乳房进行积极治疗,而是建议谨慎等待 3 个月,并再次进行乳房 X 线检查。贝丝向她的肿瘤医生表达了担忧,"那个斑点可能是癌症,3 个月后,可能开始扩散到整个乳房!"贝斯的肿瘤医生解释说,由于这个斑点在之前的乳房 X 线检查中已经稳定下来,所以不太可能是一个活跃的癌症部位。医生让她放心,在接下来的三个月里,她可以做一些事情来对抗癌症。

在观察等待期间,贝丝的抗癌计划包括消炎饮食和安全运动。她把红肉和苏打水换成了豆类、蔬菜和气泡水,并加入了一个舞蹈小组,每周锻炼三天。减肥和运动不仅改善了贝丝的身体形象,也减少了她对癌症生长或扩散的担忧,"我正在做我所能做的一切来保持健康,这让我感觉很好!"

人们在观察等待期通常会担忧,但如果注意自己的思考方式并照顾好自己,在观察等待期你可能会真正关注有意义的活动,而不是关注自己是一个癌症患者。

Unit 9

产 后 恢 复

从你生下孩子的那一刻起,你就正式成为了一个母亲。每个新妈妈在分娩后的最初几个小时的经历略有一些不同,但有一些共同的特点。

在产后初期,新妈妈还不习惯频繁地喂养婴儿,但这是来自新生儿对你和他们的健康的反馈。频繁的母乳喂养有助于刺激催产素的分泌和子宫的收缩。这样的子宫收缩称为产后阵痛。一些女性能感觉到,尤其是在哺乳期间,而另一些女性则不会。同时,这种收缩有助于使胎盘的插入点变小,这样你就可以减少失血。

若是顺产,产后你会感到会阴部位疼痛和肿胀,使用冲洗罐可以让上厕所变得更容易。冲洗罐里装上跟体温一样温度的水,用来冲洗而不是擦拭会阴部位。如果你有任何撕裂或缝线,这样做特别有用。

若是剖腹产,你可能不会有阴部疼痛和肿胀,但需要非常小心呵护切口,比如小心地走动,在哺乳时保护好切口,甚至避免走楼梯或其他会对切口造成压力的动作。因为剖腹产后的母乳喂养相对来说比较有挑战性,所以了解一些关于剖腹产后护理的技巧也很有帮助。

无论你以何种方式分娩,无论分娩的过程多么顺利,产后的前六周都是一个"恢复期"。你的身体需要一个重组的机会,所以请尽情休息,善待自己。

对于许多妇女来说,产后恶露可持续 6 周左右。在此期间,不仅身体外部有明显的恢复迹象,如失血和皮肤松弛,你的身体内部也在恢复。剖腹产手术的切口需要好几个星期才能愈合。阴道分娩撕裂或会阴切开术也需要时间才能完全愈合。婴儿通过的阴道组织本身也需要时间来恢复到接近婴儿出生前的状态。

一些女性感觉她们的身体和器官的确完全恢复到了婴儿出生前的状态,而另一些女性则感觉从未完全恢复到分娩前的状态。

每一位新妈妈,不论采用何种分娩方式,请记住,分娩后的几周应该对自己有耐心。你现在的生活不一样了。新生儿要经常护理,这有助于他们的成长。因此,你应该坐着,静养,让你的身体得到恢复。对这个过程要有耐心。你可能会觉得你什么都没做,但是从分娩和哺乳这样重大的变化中恢复过来是一件需要时间、精力和注意力的大事。

Unit 10

中　医

在中医看来,我们生活在一个万物相连的宇宙中。人体与自然有着密不可分的关系。人体本身也是一个有机整体。精神和身体并不是分开来看的。身体的一个部位发生的变化会影响身体的其他部位。

根据中国古代哲学,人类和地球上的其他生命体都是气的产物。气是控制人的精神和身体运转与运行的一种重要力量和能量。只有气血、阴阳和谐,人与自然和谐,才能保证人类的健康。否则,如果平衡被破坏,人就会受到疾病的侵袭。

为了促进气血畅通,保持身体健康,帮助预防疾病,确保快速康复,中医有多种传统的疗法,如中药,针灸、穴位敷贴、拔罐、推拿、刮痧,饮食和生活方式的改变,锻炼(通常指气功或太极)。

针灸是在经络和穴位理论的指导下进行的。它是将非常细的针插入体表下方的穴位,以减轻疼痛、治疗疾病和促进健康。

传统中医认为夏季的三伏天和冬季最冷的日子是阴阳之间的转换点。人们纷纷来到医院进行穴位敷贴,以预防呼吸道疾病、过敏性疾病、风湿性疾病和顽固性皮肤病。

虽然有些人可能很难理解中医的原理,但全世界有越来越多的人开始学习和实践中医。其良好的治疗效果和轻微的毒副作用是引起人们关注的主要原因。中医是中华文化的瑰宝,也是世界文化的瑰宝。

Unit 11

康　复　团　队

康复团队通常包括医生、护士、社会工作者、物理治疗师和作业治疗师。其他学科,如语言病理学、临床心理学、药理学或营养学,可根据需要进行咨询。

医生

专门从事康复医学的医生被称为理疗医生。大多数康复部门雇用了理疗医生。初级保健医生也可以对患者的医疗问题进行监督。

护士

护理人员对患者进行初步评估,实施康复计划,监控治疗过程,并记录患者的进展情况。他们与团队合作并确保有其他医疗问题的患者得到适当的治疗。护士强调治疗的目标和技术,向患者及家属提供教育,并负责确保护理的连续性。

物理治疗师(PTs)

物理治疗师通过专注于大肌肉运动技能来干预并帮助患者实现自我管理。比如,物理治疗师教导患者如何使用拐杖、假肢和轮椅进行移动。他们也可以教授用于执行某些日常生活活动的技术,例如转移(如进入和离开床)、走动和上厕所。物理治疗师还可以使用热敷或冷敷、超声波或电刺激来缓解患者疼痛、减轻肿胀和改善肌肉张力。

作业治疗师(OTs)

作业治疗师致力于培养患者日常生活活动所涉及的精细运动技能,例如进食、卫生和穿衣所需的技能。作业治疗师还教导患者如何运用独立的生活技能,如烹饪和购物。许多康复部门有设备齐全的公寓,患者可以在有监控的模拟环境中练习独立的生活技能。作业治疗师教授协调(例如,手部动作)及认知再训练相关的技能,从而实现这些目的。

语言病理学家(SLPs)

语言病理学家(SLPs)评估和重新训练患者的言语、语言或吞咽问题。一些患者,特别是那些经历过头部受伤或脑卒中的患者,在言语和语言方面都有困难。患有脑卒中的患者也可能有吞咽困难。语言病理学家提供吞咽困难的筛查和测试。如果患者有此问题,语言病理学家建议采用适当的食物和喂食技术。

Unit 12

将图像变成感觉以辅助盲人

几年前,科学家开始了解大脑的某些部位具有某些确定的功能。例如,一部分负责呼吸;另一部分管理嗅觉。科学家认为我们的大脑无法改变,但后来他们发现,大脑在必要时会自我重组。约瑟夫·劳斯切克是华盛顿乔治敦大学的生理学和生物物理学教授。他想知道这种改变的能力是否可以解释盲人为平衡他们的视力障碍改善了其他感官。约瑟夫·劳斯切克教授以及来自芬兰和比利时的研究人员使用 FMRI 扫描仪找到了答案。这就是功能性磁共振成像。

该机器记录了十二名盲人和十二名视力正常人执行涉及声音和触摸任务时的大脑活动。例如,他们将尝试确定声音来自哪个方向,或者哪个手指感觉到轻微的振动。劳斯切克教授说,在听觉和触觉的测试中,仅仅只有盲人大脑中的视皮质变得活跃。他说,这项研究和较早的研究促使开发了一种旨在帮助盲人的实验装置。它可以将相机拍摄的图像处理成可以被佩戴它的盲人感触到的感觉。约瑟夫·劳斯切克说:"因此,我们希望制造一种设备,该设备基本能将视觉信息转换为听觉信息,然后利用盲人大脑的惊人储备来处理声音和触觉信息。"

医学英语常用前后缀

- a-[无，缺] ▲anemia[贫血] ▲atonia[无张力] ▲asymptomatic[无症状的] ▲amenorrhea[闭经]
- ab-[分离] ▲abduct[外展] ▲abscission[切除]
- acou（acu)-[听觉] ▲acumeter[听力计] ▲acouophone[助听器]
- acro-[肢端] ▲acromegaly[肢端肥大症] ▲acromastitis[乳头炎]
- ad（af，an)-[邻近，向上] ▲adrenal[肾上腺] ▲adaxial[近轴的] ▲annexa[附件]
- -ad[……侧] ▲ventrad[向腹侧] ▲cephalad[向头侧]
- adeno-[腺] ▲adenocyte[腺细胞] ▲adenoidism[腺体病]
- adipo-[脂肪] ▲adiposis[肥胖症] ▲adiponecrosis[脂肪坏死]
- adreno-[肾上腺] ▲adrenocorticoid[肾上腺皮质激素] ▲adrenalin[肾上腺素] ▲adrenal[肾上腺]
- -aemia(emia)[血症] ▲bacteremia[菌血症] ▲leukemia[白血病]
- albi（albino)-[白色] ▲albumin[白蛋白] ▲albinism[白化病]
- -algesia[痛觉] ▲hypoalgesia[痛觉减退]
- -algia[痛] ▲arthralgia[关节痛] ▲cephalgia[头痛] ▲neuralgia[神经痛]
- alkali-[碱] ▲alkalosis[碱中毒]
- alveo-[牙槽，肺泡] ▲alveolitis[肺泡炎] ▲alveobronchiolitis[支气管肺泡炎]
- ambi-[复，双] ▲ambiopia[复视] ▲ambivert[双重性格]
- ambly-[弱] ▲amblyopia[弱视] ▲amblyaphia[触觉迟钝]
- amylo-[淀粉] ▲amyloidosis[淀粉样变] ▲amylase[淀粉酶]
- angio-[血管] ▲angiography[血管造影术] ▲angioedema[血管性水肿] ▲angeitis[脉管炎] ▲angiofibroma[血管纤维瘤]
- ante-[前] ▲antenatal[产前的] ▲anteflexion[前屈]
- antero-[前] ▲anterolateral[前侧壁] ▲anteroventral[前腹侧]
- anti-[抗，反] ▲antibiotics[抗生素] ▲antihypertensives[降压药] ▲anticoagulant[抗凝剂]
- rarchno-[蛛网膜] ▲arachnoiditis[蛛网膜炎]
- archo-[肛门，直肠] ▲archorrhagia[肛门出血] ▲archosyrinx[直肠灌注器]
- arterio-[动脉] ▲arteriospasm[动脉痉挛] ▲arteriosclerosis[动脉硬化]
- arthro-[关节] ▲arthrocentesis[关节穿刺术] ▲arthrotomy[关节切开术] ▲arthritis[关节炎]
- -ase[酶] ▲oxidase[氧化酶] ▲proteinase[蛋白酶]
- -asthenia[无力] ▲myasthenia[肌无力] ▲neurasthenia[神经衰弱]
- audio-[听力] ▲audiology[听力学] ▲audiometer[听力计]
- auto-[自己] ▲autoimmune[自身免疫的] ▲autohemotherapy[自体血疗法]
- bacilli-[杆菌] ▲bacillosis[杆菌病] ▲bacilluria[杆菌尿]
- bacterio-[细菌] ▲bacteriology[细菌学] ▲bactericide[杀菌剂]
- baro-[压力] ▲barometer[气压计] ▲baroreceptor[压力感受器]
- bary-[迟钝] ▲barylalia[言语不清] ▲baryacusia[听觉迟钝]

- bi-[双] ▲bicuspid[二尖瓣]] ▲bilateral[两侧的]
- bili-[胆汁] ▲bilirubin[胆红素]
- bio-[生命] ▲biology[生物学] ▲biopsy[活体组织检查]
- -blast[母细胞] ▲spermatoblast[精子细胞] ▲melanoblast[成黑色素细胞] ▲osteoblast[成骨细胞]
- brachy-[短] ▲brachypnea[气短] ▲brachydactylia[短指（趾）畸形]
- brady-[迟缓] ▲bradycardia[心动过缓] ▲bradypsychia[精神不振]
- broncho-[支气管] ▲bronchoscopy[支气管镜检查] ▲bronchospasm[支气管痉挛] ▲bronchitis[支气管炎]
- bronchiolo-[细支气管] ▲bronchiolectasis[细支气管扩张]
- calci-[钙] ▲calcification[钙化] ▲calcicosilicosis[钙沉着症]
- carbo-[碳] ▲carbohydrate[碳水化合物] ▲carbohaemia[碳酸血症]
- carcino-[癌] ▲carcinogen[致癌物]
- cardio-[心，贲门] ▲cardiotonics[强心剂] ▲cardioplasty[贲门成形术]
- -cele[疝，肿物] ▲omphalocele[脐膨出] ▲hysterocele[子宫脱垂] ▲ophthalmocele[眼球突出]
- celio-[腹] ▲celialgia[腹痛] ▲celioscopy[腹腔镜检查]
- -centesis[穿刺] ▲arthrocentesis[关节穿刺术] ▲abdominocentesis[腹腔穿刺]
- cephalo-[头] ▲cephaloxia[斜颈] ▲cephalopathy[头部疾病] ▲cephalotomy[穿颅术]
- cerebello-[小脑] ▲cerebellitis[小脑炎] ▲cerebellum[小脑]
- cerebro-[大脑] ▲cerebritis[大脑炎] ▲cerebrology[脑学]
- chemo-[化学] ▲chemotherapy[化疗]
- chloro-[绿，氯] ▲chloroform[氯仿] ▲chloromycetin[氯霉素] ▲chlorophyll[叶绿素]
- cholangio-[胆道] ▲cholangitis[胆管炎] ▲cholangiectasis[胆管扩张]
- cholo-[胆] ▲cholagogue[利胆剂] ▲cholelithiasis[胆石症] ▲cholecystitis[胆囊炎] ▲cholesterol[胆固醇]
- chondro-[软骨] ▲chondrosarcoma[软骨肉瘤] ▲chondrification[骨软化]
- chromo-[色素] ▲cytochrome[细胞色素] ▲chromosome[染色体]
- -cide[杀……剂] ▲germicide[杀菌剂] ▲aborticide[堕胎药]
- circum-[周围] ▲circumoral[口周的] ▲circumcision[包皮环切术]
- coagulo-[凝固] ▲coagulant[凝血药]
- colo-[结肠] ▲colotomy[结肠切开术] ▲coloptosis[结肠下垂]
- colpo（coleo)-[阴道] ▲coleospastia[阴道痉挛] ▲colposcope[阴道镜]
- contra-[反，逆] ▲contraindication[禁忌证] ▲contraceptive[避孕药]
- counter-[反，逆] ▲counteragent[反作用剂] ▲conuterpoison[解毒剂]
- cranio-[颅] ▲craniomalacia[颅骨软化] ▲cranioclasis[碎颅术]
- -cyst-[囊] ▲cystomy[膀胱切开术] ▲dacryocyst[泪囊]
- -cyte-[细胞] ▲lymphocyte[淋巴细胞] ▲cytolysis[细胞溶解]
- de-[除去] ▲detoxication[解毒]
- dento[牙] ▲dentistry[牙科学] ▲dentalgia[齿痛]
- -derm-[皮肤] ▲epiderm[表皮] ▲dermatology[皮肤病学] ▲dermoplasty[皮肤成形术]
- dextro-[右] ▲dextrocardia[右位心] ▲dexiotropic[右旋的]
- dis-[分离] ▲discission[截囊术] ▲disinfection[消毒]
- duodeno-[十二指肠] ▲duodenitis[十二指肠炎] ▲duodenostomy[十二指肠造口术]
- -dynia[痛] ▲acrodynia[肢体痛] ▲urethrodynia[尿道痛]

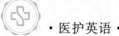

• dys-[异常] ▲dysfunction[功能紊乱] ▲dyshormonism[内分泌障碍] ▲dysuria[排尿困难]

• -ectasis[扩张] ▲gastroectasis[胃扩张] ▲aerenterectasia[肠胀气] ▲bronchiectasia[支气管扩张]

• -ectomy[切除术] ▲appendectomy[阑尾切除术] ▲lipectomy[脂肪切除术]

• -edema[水肿] ▲encephaledema[脑水肿] ▲myxedema[黏液性水肿]

• -emesia[呕] ▲hematemesis[呕血] ▲helminthemesia[吐虫]

• encephalo-[脑] ▲encephaloma[脑瘤] ▲encephaledema[脑水肿]

• endo-[内] ▲endocarditis[心内膜炎] ▲endoscope[内窥镜]

• entero-[肠] ▲enteritis[小肠炎] ▲enterovirus[肠病毒]

• epi-[上,外] ▲epigastrium[上腹部]

• erythro-[红] ▲erythromycin[红霉素] ▲erythroderma[红皮病]

• esophago-[食管] ▲esophagoscope[食管镜] ▲esophagitis[食管炎]

• extra-[……外] ▲extracellular[细胞外的] ▲extrasystole[额外收缩]

• facio-[面] ▲facioplegia[面瘫] ▲facioplasty[面部成形术]

• -fast[耐] ▲acid-fast[抗酸的] ▲uviofast[耐紫外线的]

• febri-[热] ▲febricula[低热] ▲febrifacient[产热的]

• feti-[胎儿] ▲feticulture[妊娠期卫生] ▲fetometry[胎儿测量法]

• fibro-[纤维] ▲fibroblast[成纤维细胞] ▲fibrosis[纤维化]

• fore-[前] ▲forebrain[前脑] ▲forehead[前额]

• -form[形状] ▲oviform[卵形的] ▲granuliform[颗粒状的]

• fungi-[真菌,霉菌] ▲fungicide[杀真菌剂] ▲fungistasis[制霉菌作用]

• gastro-[胃] ▲gastroptosis[胃下垂] ▲gastroenteritis[肠胃炎] ▲gastroscopy[胃镜检查] ▲gastratrophy[胃萎缩]

• -gen[原,剂] ▲glycogen[糖原] ▲pathogen[病原体] ▲androgen[雄激素] ▲estrogen[雌激素]

• -genic[……性] ▲cardiogenic[心源性的] ▲allergenic[变应反应]

• giganto-[巨大] ▲gigantocyte[巨红细胞] ▲gigantism[巨人症]

• gingivo-[牙龈] ▲gingivitis[牙龈炎] ▲gingivostomatitis[龈口炎]

• glosso-[舌] ▲glossoplegia[舌瘫痪]

• gluco-[糖] ▲glucoprotein[糖蛋白] ▲glucocorticoid[糖皮质激素]

• glyco-[糖] ▲glycogen[糖原] ▲glycosuria[糖尿]

• -grade[级,度] ▲centigrade[摄氏温度计] ▲retrograde[逆行性]

• -gram[克,图] ▲microgram[微克] ▲electroencephalogram[脑电图]

• -graph(y)[……仪(法)] ▲electrocardiogram[心电图] ▲bronchography[支气管造影术]

• gyneco-[妇女] ▲gynecology[妇科学] ▲gynecopathy[妇科病]

• hemo(hemato)-[血] ▲hemoglobin[血红蛋白] ▲hematoma[血肿]

• hemi-[半] ▲hemiplegia[偏瘫] ▲hemicrania[偏头病]

• hepato-[肝] ▲hepatitis[肝炎] ▲hepatocirrhosis[肝硬化] ▲hepatosplenomegaly[肝脾大]

• hidro-[汗] ▲hyperhidrosis[多汗症] ▲anhidrosis[无汗症]

• histo-[组织] ▲histology[组织学] ▲histomorphology[组织形态学]

• holo-[全] ▲holonarcosis[全麻] ▲holoenzyme[全酶]

• homo-[同] ▲homotype[同型] ▲homologue[同系物] ▲homoplasty[同种移植术]

• hydro-[水] ▲hydropericardium[心包积液] ▲hydrolysis[水解]

• hypr-[高] ▲hypercalcemia[高钙血症] ▲hyperthyroidism[甲状腺功能亢进]

• hypno-[睡眠] ▲hypnotics[安眠药] ▲hypnotherapy[催眠疗法]

- hypo-[低] ▲hypotension[低血压] ▲hypoglycemia[低血糖]
- hystero-[子宫] ▲hysterospasm[子宫绞痛] ▲hysteroptosis[子宫下垂]
- -ia[病] ▲melancholia[忧郁症] ▲pyrexia[发热]
- -iatrics[医学] ▲pediatrics[儿科学] ▲geriatrics[老年医学]
- -iatry[医学] ▲psychiatry[精神病学] ▲pediatry[儿科学]
- immuno-[免疫] ▲immunoglobulin[免疫球蛋白] ▲immunotherapy[免疫疗法]
- infra-[下] ▲infraorbital[眶下的] ▲infrared[红外线的]
- inter-[间] ▲intervertebral[椎间的] ▲intercellular[细胞间的]
- intra-[内] ▲intravenous[静脉内的] ▲intracranial[颅内的] ▲intramuscular[肌肉内的]
- -ist[家] ▲pathologist[病理学家] ▲anatomist[解剖学家]
- -itis[炎症] ▲cellulitis[蜂窝织炎] ▲myocarditis[心肌炎]
- leuco (leuko)-[白] ▲leucorrhea[白带] ▲leukocytosis[白细胞增多] ▲leukemia[白血病]
- lipo-(脂) ▲lipotrophy[脂肪增多] ▲lipase[脂肪酶]
- -lith[结石] ▲cholelith[胆结石] ▲cholelithiasis[胆石症]
- -logy[学] ▲terminology[术语] ▲cardiology[心脏病学]
- lumbo-[腰] ▲lumbosacral[腰骶部的] ▲lumbago[腰痛] ▲lumbodynia[腰痛]
- lympho-[淋巴] ▲lymphedema[淋巴水肿] ▲lymphocytopenia[淋巴细胞减少症]
- -lysis(lytic)[松解,分解] ▲aythrolysis[关节松解术] ▲spasmolytic[解痉的]
- macro-[大] ▲macrophage[巨噬细胞] ▲macromolecule[大分子]
- mal-[不良] ▲malnutrition[营养不良] ▲malfunction[功能不全]
- -megaly[巨大] ▲cardiomegaly[心脏肥大] ▲cephalomegaly[巨头畸形]
- meningo-[脑膜] ▲meningitis[脑膜炎] ▲meningoencephalitis[脑膜脑炎]
- meno-[月经] ▲dysmenorrhea[痛经] ▲menopause[绝经]
- -meter[表,计] ▲spirometer[肺活量计] ▲pyrometer[高温计]
- -metry[测量法] ▲iodometry[碘定量法]
- micro-[小] ▲micropump[微型泵] ▲microliter[微升]
- mono-[单-] ▲mononucleosis[单核细胞增多] ▲monomer[单体]
- multi-[多] ▲multinuclear[多核的] ▲multipara[经产妇]
- myelo-[髓] ▲myelocele[脊髓膨出] ▲myelocyte[髓细胞]
- myo-[肌] ▲myocarditis[心肌炎] ▲myofibroma[肌纤维瘤]
- naso-[鼻] ▲nasoscope[鼻镜] ▲nasitis[鼻炎]
- neo-[新] ▲neoplasm[新生物] ▲neomycin[新霉素]
- nephro-[肾] ▲nephropathy[肾病] ▲nephrosclerosis[肾硬变]
- neuro-[神经] ▲neuroma[神经瘤] ▲neurodermatitis[神经性皮炎]
- non-[非] ▲non-electrolyte[非电解质] ▲nonfatal[非致命的]
- nulli-[无] ▲nullipara[未产妇] ▲nulligravida[未孕妇]
- nutri-[营养] ▲nutrition[营养] ▲nutrology[营养学]
- oculo-[眼] ▲oculist[眼科医生] ▲oculus dexter[右眼] ▲oculus sinister[左眼]
- oligo-[少] ▲oligophrenia[智力发育不全] ▲oliguria[少尿]
- -oma[肿瘤] ▲adenoma[腺瘤] ▲osteoma[骨瘤]
- onco-[肿瘤] ▲oncology[肿瘤学] ▲oncogene[癌基因]
- ophthalmo-[眼] ▲ophthalmocele[眼球突出] ▲ophthalmoplegia[眼肌麻痹]
- -osis[病] ▲cirrhosis[肝硬化] ▲mycosis[霉菌病]
- osteo-[骨] ▲osteomalacia[骨软化] ▲osteoarthritis[骨关节炎]

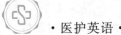

- oto-[耳] ▲otolith[耳石] ▲otoplasty[耳成形术] ▲otopyosis[耳化脓]
- pan-[全] ▲panimmunity[多种免疫] ▲pantalgia[身痛] ▲pantatrophia[全身营养不良]
- -para[产妇] ▲primipara[初产妇] ▲nullipara[未产妇]
- -pathy[病] ▲dermatopathy[皮肤病] ▲cardiomyopathy[心肌病]
- pedia-[儿童] ▲pediatrician[儿科医师] ▲pediatrics[儿科学]
- -penia[减少] ▲leucopenia[白细胞减少症] ▲thrombopenia[血小板减少]
- per-[经] ▲percutaneous[经皮的]
- peri-[周围] ▲pericarditis[心包炎] ▲perianal[肛周的]
- pharmaco-[药] ▲pharmacokinetics[药代动力学]
- physio-[物理] ▲physiotheraphy[理疗] ▲physicochemistry[物理化学]
- -plasty[成形术] ▲angioplasty[血管成形术] ▲homoplasty[同种移植] ▲gastroplasty[胃成形术]
- -plegia[瘫] ▲paraplegia[截瘫] ▲hemiplegia[偏瘫]
- pleuro-[胸膜] ▲pleuritis[胸膜炎] ▲pleurocentesis[胸腔穿刺术]
- -pnea[呼吸] ▲orthopnea[端坐呼吸] ▲tachypnea[呼吸急促]
- pneumo-[气,肺] ▲pneumothorax[气胸] ▲pneumococcus[肺炎球菌]
- poly-[多] ▲polyuria[多尿] ▲polycholia[胆汗过多]
- post-[后] ▲postpartum[产后] ▲postoperation[术后]
- pre-[前] ▲premenopause[绝经前期] ▲premature[早产] ▲preload[前负荷]
- pseudo-[假] ▲pseudohypertrophy[假性肥大] ▲pseudomembranous[假膜的]
- psycho-[精神,心理] ▲psychology[心理学] ▲psychiatry[精神病学]
- -ptosis[下垂] ▲nephroptosis[肾下垂] ▲hysteroptosis[子宫下垂]
- -ptysis[咯] ▲pyoptysis[咯脓] ▲hemoptysis[咯血]
- pyo-[脓] ▲pyorrhea[溢脓] ▲pyosis[化脓]
- radio-[放射] ▲radiotherapy[放射治疗] ▲radiology[放射学]
- recto-[直肠] ▲rectitis[直肠炎] ▲rectectomy[直肠切除术]
- retino-[视网膜] ▲retinitis[视网膜炎] ▲retinodialysis[视网膜分离]
- rhino-[鼻] ▲rhinitis[鼻炎] ▲rhinorrhea[鼻漏]
- -rrhagia[出血] ▲gastorrhagia[胃出血] ▲hemorrhage[出血] ▲pneumorrhagia[肺出血]
- -rrhaphy[缝合术] ▲neurorrhaphy[神经缝合术] ▲salpingorrhaphy[输卵管缝合术]
- -rrhea[流出] ▲diarrhea[腹泻] ▲menorrhea[月经]
- schisto-[裂] ▲schistosomiasis[血吸虫病] ▲schistoglossia[舌裂]
- scirrho-[硬] ▲scirrhosarca[硬皮病] ▲scirrhoma[硬癌]
- sclero-[硬] ▲scleroderma[硬皮病] ▲sclerometer[硬度计]
- -scope(scopy)[镜,检查] ▲stethoscope[听诊器] ▲otoscope[耳镜] ▲proctoscopy[直肠镜检查]
- semi-[半] ▲semicoma[半昏迷] ▲semiliquid[半流体]
- spondylo-[脊椎] ▲spondylopathy[脊椎病] ▲spondylitis[脊椎炎]
- -stomy[造口术] ▲colostomy[结肠造口术] ▲ilecolostomy[回结肠吻合术]
- sub-[下,亚] ▲subacute[亚急性的] ▲subabdominal[下腹部的]
- super-[在……上] ▲superficial[浅的] ▲superoxide[超氧化物]
- supra-[上] ▲supraventricular[室上性的] ▲suprarenalism[肾上腺机能亢进]
- tachy-[快] ▲tachycardia[心动过速] ▲tachypnea[呼吸急促]
- -therapy[治疗] ▲massotherapy[按摩治疗] ▲pharmacotherapy[药物治疗]

• thermo-[热] ▲thermometer[温度计] ▲thermatology[热疗学]

• thrombo-[血栓，血小板] ▲ thrombolysis[溶栓] ▲ thrombocytopenia[血小板减少症] ▲thrombosis[血栓形成]

• -tomy[切开术] ▲tracheotomy[气管切开术] ▲ovariotomy[卵巢切开术]

• tracheo-[气管] ▲tracheoscope[气管镜] ▲tracheorrhagia[气管出血]

• trans-[经,转移] ▲transurethral[经尿道] ▲transfusion[输血]

• -trophy[营养] ▲dystrophy[营养不良] ▲atrophy[萎缩]

• ultra-[超过] ▲ultraviolet[紫外线] ▲ultrasound[超声]

• utero-[子宫] ▲uteroscope[子宫镜] ▲uterotonic[子宫收缩药]

• vaso-[血管] ▲vasomotion[血管舒缩] ▲vasodilator[血管扩张药]

参考文献
CANKAOWENXIAN

[1] 江晓东,晏柳清,谢家鑫.医护英语入门教程[M].2版.武汉:华中科技大学出版社,2013.

[2] 徐小贞.新职业英语:行业篇[M].2版.北京:外语教学与研究出版社,2015.

[3] Lin J.涉外护理英语:情境对话[M].北京:外语教学与研究出版社,2006.

[4] 刘军,杨明星,章学文.医学英语[M].郑州:郑州大学出版社,2014.

[5] 医护英语水平考试办公室.全国医护英语水平考试考试大纲:全新版[M].北京:高等教育出版社,2017.

[6] 唐巧英,罗渝,刘韬.医护英语[M].北京:人民卫生出版社,2014.

[7] 雷慧.实用医院英语[M].2版.北京:人民卫生出版社,2014.

[8] 教育部《医学英语》教材编写组.医学英语[M].北京:高等教育出版社,2001.

[9] 刘红霞.护理专业英语[M].北京:中国中医药出版社,2013.